With the Help of Our Friends from France

Stabilizing and Living with Advanced Breast Cancer

SECOND EDITION

Best Wishes to everyone at the Women Care — Carol

Carol Silverander

This book is not intended to be, nor should it be, used as a substitute for professional medical care. It is intended, instead, to aid patients in becoming active participants in their own treatment and to work more closely with their physicians and health care team.

With the Help of Our Friends from France

Stabilizing and Living with Advanced Breast Cancer

First Edition 2005
Second Edition 2007

ISBN 0-976-83161-9
Library of Congress Registration Number TX 6-247-956

CMS
PRESS

616 E. Cota Street, Santa Barbara, CA 93103
Copies of this book may be ordered at www.cmspress.com

PRINTED IN THE UNITED STATES OF AMERICA

DEDICATION

There are two people who have been closer to me than life itself—my twin sister Cheryl Karp and my husband Michael Silverander. I don't know how I would have been able to get through my struggle with cancer without their amazing love and support. This book has only been possible because of their encouragement and their confidence. Cheryl and Michael spent many hours reading and re-reading the numerous drafts of this book. It was Michael who not only did all of the editing of this book, which helped it flow much better than it would have, but he in particular helped me grasp the technical information about endobiogénie. I so appreciate how much time he spent with me sifting through the data, and for designing this book. Both Cheryl and Michael have given me the strength I have needed to continue to fight the fight. This book is for them.

Acknowledgements

Many people have been instrumental in the creation of this book. First, I want to thank my doctors, without whom I would almost certainly not be here today. My oncologist, Dr. Thomas Woliver, was the first doctor I saw after cancer metastasized in my liver. Through his gentle caring, he gave me hope that I could live with cancer. This hope sustained me through the treatments I would have to endure. I am grateful to him for openly accepting my desire to check out complementary treatments that would enhance traditional chemotherapy. Through seemingly endless emails, he reviewed my written explanations of all the medical procedures I have gone through, and told me if they were correct. His help has been invaluable.

My deepest gratitude also goes to the incredible Dr. Jean-Claude Lapraz. He helped me to understand my body much better than I had ever thought possible. His insights allowed me to make sense of the cancer and realize how outside influences like stress can effect the body's ability to fight disease. Dr. Lapraz encouraged me to write this book. He felt that reading about my experiences would help others. These two amazing physicians, as well as Dr. Christian Duraffourd, transformed my life. I don't know how I can ever repay them. My medical team was rounded out by a wonderful chiropractor, Dr. Thomas Rook. He not only made adjustments to my body, helping it become strong and correcting aliments such as carpal tunnel syndrome, but also has been a great source of emotional support.

Through Dr. Lapraz I met Patrice Pauly, the dedicated and talented individual who translated my book from English to French. Patrice educated me more completely about the methods of Drs. Lapraz and Duraffourd, sending a complete explanation of endobiogénie when this book was in its infancy. It was only then that I fully understood how Dr. Lapraz's treatments had been helping me for several years. Patrice also has been a very valuable editor and friend. All of the help he so willingly and unselfishly gave made this book much better than it would have been otherwise.

I also want to thank my yoga buddies—Chris, Katarina, Elaine, Carolyn, Corinne, Alice, Ruth, Eileen and all of the others who have come and gone. They have been an inspiration to me, as I've watched them battle their own cancers with such amazing courage. And, many thanks to the yoga teachers at the Cancer Center of Santa Barbara—Cheri, Kat, Anne, and Scott—for helping all of us strengthen our minds and bodies after the abuse they received in fighting our disease.

A special thank you goes to Angela Rooney, who first told me how to get in touch with Dr. Lapraz. Without her, this journey could not have been possible. And, also to Angela Barbero for her careful and thoughtful proof-reading.

There are many others I want to thank for taking the time to read my manuscript and for giving me their valuable feedback: Colin Nicholls, Danny Pauly, Christa Gyssels, Daniela Welteke, Cindy Silverglat, Chris Dahl, Jane Gottlieb, Cheri Clampett, Christine Nevet, Dr. Marta Ketchel and Dr. Robert Schwebel. My gratitude also goes to Tu-Vi Luong and Dr. Kathleen Zisser for helping me to understand more thoroughly how acupuncture helps bring balance to the body. I must also mention the amazing and dedicated people at the Endobiogenic Integrative Medical Center in Pocatello, Idaho who are responsible for bringing endobiogénie to the United States: Annemarie Buhler, Eric and Annette Davis, Elisabeth "Nica" George, Dr. Jean Bokelmann and Amy Humpherys. Thanks also to Antoine Codet Boisse for helping me to understand the Biology of Functions.

I must also give a special acknowledgment to the nurses in the chemo room at the Cancer Center of Santa Barbara for their loving care and support. Their amazing kindness and cheerful attitude made my treatments so much easier!

And Finally to my incredible family—my children Michael and Kim Romano and David Silverander, my sister Nancy Davison, my brother-in-law Leonard Karp, my brother Vernon and daughter-in-law Lisa Romano—all of you were there to help me get through my battle with cancer, and also took the time to read my book and listen to what I had to say. Your suggestions were honest and invaluable—my love goes out to each of you.

CONTENTS

Introduction

When I was told that cancer had spread from my breast to my liver, and that I had only a three percent chance of beating it, I knew I was going to be in for the battle of my life. The oncologist who was my doctor at the time said she thought I would be able to live for two years. That was a very frightening thought—there was still a lot of living I wanted to do.

Now, eight years after receiving that news, I am being treated by a forward-thinking oncologist and another, quite unique physician from Paris, France. While the cancer remains in my liver, my condition is stable and my general health is excellent. The cancer does not restrict my life in any way, and those who meet me—particularly medical professionals—are astounded to learn that I have fourth-stage breast cancer.

I credit this most unusual outcome to the therapies—both conventional and complementary—that I have been fortunate enough to receive. I have been able to take advantage of recent advances in chemotherapy with drugs that are both less toxic and more effective than those previously available. I have also benefited hugely from the treatments prescribed by my doctor in Paris. Over the past 30 years, he and his colleagues have developed a very thorough diagnostic and therapeutic tool called endo-biogénie. Through the use of extensive blood analysis and a thorough clinical examination they are able to determine where imbalances exist in the body—imbalances that eventually lead to disease. They prescribe treatments including plant-based medicines and changes in diet in order to correct these imbalances. This, in turn, can help prevent and halt the spread of disease.

For me, this has meant that my cancer has been stopped in its tracks. The tumors in my liver are stable and have not spread to other parts of my body. I have also been able to achieve and maintain a remarkable state of good health. I have never felt better or had more energy at any time in my life. It is important to note that my doctor in Paris believes that his treatments should complement conventional cancer therapies—not replace them. He believes it is crucial that he and my oncologist work together in treating my disease.

Now, recent developments have brought endobiogénie to the United States. Those interested in this diagnostic and therapeutic tool can complement conventional treatments by going no further than Pocatello, Idaho instead of traveling to Paris. Details on the Endobiogenic Integrative Medical Center in Pocatello can be found in the resources section at the end of this book.

I have learned many things since I was first diagnosed with stage-one breast cancer in December, 1997. If I had known then what I know now, I would have done many things differently. My story shows how my view of cancer changed as I opened up and came to accept the diagnosis, but not the prognosis. Hopefully, those who read this book will benefit from my experiences. I especially hope it will encourage those battling cancer to be proactive in their own care. I hope they will inform themselves and ask questions about their treatments instead of blindly accepting them. We are, after all, our own best advocates. And, when the diagnosis is cancer, our own lives are on the line.

I feel that attitudes about treating cancer must change. I have found ways to live with my disease—in much the same way a diabetic lives with diabetes. As cancer patients change the way they view their disease, the quality of their lives will also change. Personally, I plan to live life to the fullest for many more years. I am not waiting for a miracle cure. I hope those who read my story will be inspired to never, ever give up the fight.

"Challenges make you discover things about yourself that you never really knew. They're what make the instrument stretch—what make you go beyond the norm."

—CICELY TYSON

CHAPTER ONE

The News

It was December 1999. I remember the conversation with my husband Michael as if it were yesterday! I heard him tell me that my oncologist had just called and told him that my cancer had spread from my breast to my liver. Then I just remember him crying as we held each other. I tried consoling him, but I was numb. The oncologist had called him at his office, asking if he wanted to give me the news or have her do it. He told her he would do it, and have me call her afterwards. Michael and I spoke in his conference room and he did his best to tell me everything the doctor had said.

But I needed to call the oncologist and hear it firsthand. She told me that most people whose cancer had spread like mine would live for two years. She said she hoped I could stay stable for four years, and that maybe in that time a cure for cancer would be found. When I asked about my odds of being cured, she said that three percent of people with cancer like mine actually conquer it. Wow, what a mouthful! I remember hearing those odds and thinking that someone had to be in the three percent—so why not me?

As I write this, it has been eight years since I learned the cancer had spread. Today my cancer is stable, any my treatments continue. While the tumors are still present in my liver and I have not been cured, the tumors are stable in size and my liver function is normal. The general state of my health is excellent, and I feel great. Most people I meet wonder how this is possible. Although no one has found a cure for cancer—as my oncologist hoped might happen—some new treatments have been developed, and peoples' attitudes about living with cancer have started to change.

Many of the things I hope to share in the story of my struggle may help others who have been diagnosed with cancer to live fuller and more complete lives. I have benefited from conventional treatments including chemotherapy and radiation, as well as from newer medications that weren't available when I was first diagnosed. I have also been fortunate enough to take advantage of innovative and, I feel, very effective complementary treatments involving plant-based medications. Those treatments were prescribed by a physician in Paris, France and are based on a new approach to medicine called endobiogénie. I will discuss in detail endobiogénie as it applies to cancer, and describe the changes in the state of my overall health as my body gradually returned to balance. More than anything else, I have learned a great deal, both about myself and about my disease. If, when first diagnosed, I had known what I know now, I would have managed my care in a very different manner. I hope that others will be able to benefit from my experiences.

So, how does one take the news that they have advanced cancer? I, for one, automatically went into survival mode. I was extremely calm—there was no time to reflect on the gravity of the situation. Everyone handles difficult news differently—there is no right or wrong way. I have learned that, for me, it's best to just feel the feelings and then let them go. I have also discovered that I need to be an active participant in my treatment. It doesn't matter if you have the best cancer specialists in the world working with you. It's still your life, and you need to be the one who ultimately determines the course of your treatments.

I have come to think of my cancer as a chronic illness. That means that I think in terms of treating it rather than curing it. I was lucky enough to first grasp this concept while going through intravenous chemotherapy shortly after the cancer had metastasized. Then, a few years later, in 2003, I read an article in *The Wall Street Journal* by Tara Parker-Pope that explains this idea quite well. She said:

> *"For years, doctors and patients have accepted that certain health problems, such as diabetes or heart disease, are chronic illnesses that can't be cured. The diseases are serious and life-threatening, but patients rarely view them as an immediate death sentence. Instead, they spend their final years or decades managing their disease, dutifully taking high-blood pressure pills, insulin treatments and other drugs—and living their lives. Why should cancer be any different?"*

That is my mindset, and I hope many others with cancer will come to share this point of view.

My cancer did not start at stage four. I was originally diagnosed with stage one breast cancer on New Year's Eve, 1997 at the age of 51. That was two years before we discovered the cancer had spread to my liver. It all started when my hand accidentally brushed over my left breast and I felt a lump. It felt so weird. Even though there was a lump on my breast, I didn't think of cancer. I had recently seen my gynecologist and, as always, she had given me a very thorough breast exam. When I asked Michael to see what he could feel, he said it was definitely a lump and that I should have it checked out. I decided to wait a week to see if it went away, thinking that maybe it was just a cyst. When it didn't go away after several days, I called my gynecologist. She told me it was time for my yearly mammogram anyway and that I should immediately schedule one. But, she added that it was probably nothing since she had just examined me herself and hadn't felt anything during the exam.

The mammogram was scheduled at a local hospital. The heat in the examining room wasn't working and I remember that I was so cold, sitting there naked from the waist up in my gown. They also did a sonogram. I asked why, since that had never been part of my routine annual exam. They said that the radiologist felt it was needed. Since then, I have learned why a sonogram is used as a diagnostic test. It can detect if a lump is solid or filled with fluid (which usually indicates a benign cyst). It can also show if there are irregular borders on the lump, suggesting a malignant lesion. Regular borders suggest a benign lesion. Through a sonogram, doctors can also learn about the nature of the lesion itself. Whether a lesion transmits echoes or reflects them can be an indicator of malignancy. A sonogram is also referred to as an ultrasound exam. An ultrasound technologist spreads a warm transmitting gel over the areas of the body to be scanned (which felt good because I was so cold that day) and then runs a wand-like instrument lightly through the gel. A video screen displays a moving image of the area being examined and the image is photographed for analysis. I remember being worried because the technician seemed concerned about a spot on my other breast, in addition to the area where I had felt the lump.

It seemed like forever before my doctor finally called with the results from the mammogram and sonogram. More than a week after the tests, I finally received the much anticipated telephone call, and the news was not good. The doctor told me I needed to have the tumor in my left breast surgically removed regardless of whether it was benign or malignant. She said that a needle biopsy would not be good enough—the tumor had to be removed and tested.

This presented a problem. I was living in Santa Barbara, California, but I had previously lived in Tucson, Arizona for many years. All of my doctors were there, including the gynecologist who was telling me I needed surgery. Even after moving to Santa Barbara, I had continued to see my old doctors in Tucson. It had always been easy to get my yearly exam when I visited my sisters, Cheryl (my identical twin) and Nancy. I had been seeing those same doctors in Tucson for nearly 20 years.

After hearing that I needed surgery, I called Cheryl and told her what the doctor had said. She and her husband, Len, had a close friend who is an anesthesiologist at Cedars Sinai Hospital in Los Angeles—which is only 90 miles from Santa Barbara. She said she would call him at home and get a referral for a surgeon in Southern California. He was wonderfully caring and said there was only one surgeon he would want his wife to see if she had breast cancer. He said he would have an appointment made for me for the next day. He not only made the appointment, but met Michael and me at the surgeon's office in Los Angeles to personally introduce us. I brought the x-rays that had been taken in Santa Barbara so the surgeon could examine them. He was very nice and told me that although the x-rays were of very poor quality, he could tell by the written report that this was indeed very serious. He said he suspected that the tumor would be malignant. Still, he reminded us that it was impossible to know for sure until it was taken out and tested. He also told me that the sonogram showed my other breast was free of tumors.

The surgeon said that the tumor could be removed in an outpatient procedure performed in the surgical suite in his office. We confirmed that the surgery would be covered by our medical insurance, and it was scheduled for 7:00 am the next morning—which was New Year's Eve. Our friend, the anesthesiologist who had recommended the surgeon, would administer the anesthesia. The surgeon described the procedure. After surgery, I would wake up and learn the results. If the tumor was malignant, I would have to come back a couple of days later for a second surgery where more tissue surrounding the tumor would be removed. At this time, lymph nodes would also be taken from under my arm and tested to see if the cancer had spread. Our first appointment finished with the doctor showing us photographs of mastectomies and breast reconstructions that he had performed. He told us that a mastectomy would be necessary if the tissue surrounding the tumor was shown to contain cancerous cells. It really was all very overwhelming.

Michael and I left his office and stopped at a restaurant in Los Angeles for dinner. We talked about what the doctor said. I really couldn't eat, for I was very nervous. I was still surprised about the possibility of cancer. I had been a vegetarian for the previous ten years, didn't drink and didn't smoke. There was no history of cancer in my family. In fact, I had only been in the hospital once in my entire life—for an emergency appendectomy many years earlier.

I remember saying to Michael at dinner that I thought the tumor may have been a result of my taking a hormone replacement drug (consisting of estrogen and progestin) about a year before. Although I had never had hot flashes, my gynecologist in Tucson insisted that I take the drug. She was concerned about osteoporosis, since my mother had had it, and told me the hormone replacement tablets would be good for my heart as well. A blood test was never ordered to determine if I was actually low in estrogen and progesterone. Several years later, a blood test showed that my body had an overabundance of estrogen and progesterone, and that the last thing I needed was to take more of it. Today a great deal more is known about the dangers of synthetic hormone replacement drugs than in 1996. I hope that gynecologists now will perform a blood test before prescribing such drugs for their patients. I also hope that patients will take an active role in their own care and ask for tests to confirm that hormone replacement drugs are really needed before they take them. I will talk more about hormone replacement therapy later in the book.

As we drove back to Santa Barbara that night, I called Cheryl on my cell phone to go over everything we had heard and to prepare her for the worst. She wanted to fly out immediately, but I told her to wait until we really knew if the tumor was malignant or not. If it was, she could fly out for the second surgery. I asked her to call our sister Nancy, and our brother Vernon to give them the news. I just wasn't up for explaining everything all over again. I felt that it would be better to wait for the second surgery before worrying the rest of the family.

The next morning we needed to start the drive to Los Angeles very early. The alarm sounded at 4:00 am, but we really didn't need it, as we had slept very little. So much was happening at such an accelerated pace. We took our showers and were out the door by 5:15. We reached the doctor's office before the morning rush hour traffic, checked in, and soon I found myself being prepped for the surgery.

A major part of any surgery is the anesthesia, and I was lucky to have one of the best anesthesiologists to be found anywhere. He used a very advanced technique that allowed me to awake in the operating room as soon as the procedure was over. I walked into the recovery room on my own, where I felt good enough to have a donut and coffee. Painkillers and anesthesia had always made me sick to my stomach, so this was a minor miracle.

We didn't have to wait long before results came back from the lab showing that the tumor was malignant. I had the big "C." Freshly bandaged from the surgery, I was sent across the street to see yet another doctor. This one was an internist, who was to examine me and make sure I was strong enough to withstand the second surgery, during which I would be put under a much deeper anesthesia. I received a chest x-ray, an EKG and a general physical exam. It was all quite strange, since I was freshly bandaged from the surgery that had taken place just a couple of hours before. I passed the tests with flying colors and the second surgery was scheduled for 7:30 am two days later—January 2, 1998.

We drove back to Santa Barbara and I insisted on stopping by the offices of my greeting card company so I could show my office staff that I was really okay. They were like family to me. It wasn't until then that I realized I had not called Cheryl after the surgery. When I reached her she was very upset and had been crying with worry. I felt horrible. She told me she would be on a flight the next day. She would stay with her son, Scott, who lives in Los Angeles, and then meet us at the doctor's office before the second surgery. She then planned to come back to Santa Barbara with us for the weekend. I totally understood how she was feeling. I knew I would have been exactly the same if she was having surgery. Sometimes, I think that cancer is harder on those closest to us, for they so badly want to be able to do something but are left feeling helpless. I, for one, would rather be fighting the disease than watching a member of my family deal with it.

Everyone close to me wanted to be there for the second surgery—including my sister Nancy, and my two grown children, Michael and Kim. But I really didn't want so many people around, and told them that I would call them after the surgery. In retrospect, I think that I should have allowed them to come, so they would have been able to see with their own eyes that I was really okay. My son, Michael, had just finished law school in Oregon. Kim had recently completed her undergraduate studies at UC Santa Cruz and was deciding what to do with her life. My stepson, David, was a freshman in high school, and lived with us half of the time, so he was there during all of it. It was very difficult for David, and it brought up fears that his own mother could get cancer, since the disease had been very prevalent in her family.

As I mentioned, during the second surgery more tissue would be taken from the area around where the tumor had been. The outside portions of this tissue (called the margins) would then be tested to see if they were clear of cancer cells. If the margins were clear, there would be no more surgery. If they were not, the entire breast would be removed. Additionally, during this surgery, the surgeon would remove several lymph nodes from around my left breast and from under my left arm.

These lymph nodes would also be tested to see if they contained cancerous cells. If the cancer had already spread, it would have traveled through my body's lymphatic system. If they tested clear, it was likely that the cancer had been caught before it metastasized. The treatments that would follow the surgery depended on the test results.

The surgery went smoothly and, once again, I awoke in the operating room and walked to the recovery room. I was sore under my left arm where the lymph nodes had been taken, and I was bandaged up tighter than before. Cheryl, Michael and I were sitting in the recovery room when the surgeon came in and told us he had been able to get eight lymph nodes to send to the lab for testing. I remember thinking that eight sounded like a good number. But I had no clue as to what a really appropriate number might be. Several years later I learned that eight was a rather low number. Fifteen would have been more like it, and some doctors might have taken 25 (the recommended number I have found in research is from 10-30). At the time, though, I felt very fortunate to have such a well respected surgeon. We trusted him completely and didn't question anything he said. We never felt the need for a second opinion, since he was considered one of the top breast cancer surgeons in Southern California. One reason that some surgeons take a lower number of lymph nodes is concern about causing lymphedema, a chronic swelling of the arm.

Today, there is another method that has proven very effective in determining if cancer has spread into the lymph nodes. It is called a sentinel node biopsy, and it allows doctors to determine if the cancer has spread by removing only one or two lymph nodes (instead of the 10 to 30 that would normally be taken for testing). In this procedure, a radioactive tracer and/or blue dye is injected into the region of the tumor. The dye or radioactive material is carried by the lymphatic vessels to "sentinel nodes," the first lymph nodes in line from the tumor, and the ones most likely to contain a metastasis if the cancer has spread. Usually one to three sentinel nodes are taken. Studies done at the Mayo Clinic indicate that if the sentinel node is cancer free, no further surgery is necessary. There is some question as to whether or not people whose sentinel nodes test positive for cancer cells should have further lymph nodes removed and tested, or just proceed with chemotherapy and/or hormone therapy. It should also be noted that it is sometimes difficult to find a sentinel node, and that there is some concern about the reliability of this method of diagnosis. I know one breast cancer patient who was lucky when his surgeon decided to take more lymph nodes than just the sentinel node. In his case, the sentinel node was clear and another node contained cancer cells. So, the jury is still out as to the safest method of determining if cancer has spread.

We returned home the afternoon after my second surgery. It was Friday, and I was scheduled to come back on Monday to learn the test results. We all had a lot on our minds, but everyone wanted to remain positive and not think about the possibility of the cancer having spread. Monday couldn't come soon enough for me, and that morning we sped to Los Angeles to get the results. Michael had always been in the examining room with me whenever I had seen the surgeon, but this time he stayed in the waiting room with Cheryl. I should have asked both of them to come in with me, but I didn't realize that the doctor would give me the test results there in the examining room. If possible, it's a good idea to have someone with you at all doctors' appointments. They can take notes and help you accurately remember the information that the doctor gives you. It is an emotional time and important advice can be missed.

Fortunately, the news was good for me that day—no spread of the cancer. The margins of the tissue and the eight lymph nodes were clear. The doctor told me he felt I had saved my own life, and that years later I would see this as merely a bump in the road. He predicted that I would go on to live a completely normal life. I decided to do exactly that—go on as though I had never had cancer at all. Cheryl took a flight home from Los Angeles that afternoon and we drove back to Santa Barbara.

I couldn't wait to get to my office and tell everyone that all was well. So, we stopped there on the way home and I dished out the good news. I was very sore from the surgery and felt exhausted, so after a few minutes we went home for me to rest. It had been only a week since I was first told the tumor needed to be removed. I had been on an emotional roller coaster—it all seemed so unreal.

Michael and I went back to Los Angeles several times during that next week so the surgeon could drain fluids from the incision to allow for better healing of the wound. After the first of these appointments, he placed a simple bandage over the incision. I could wear a bra over the bandage, and I began to feel normal again. Then, at the next appointment, in addition to changing the bandage, he wrapped my entire chest tightly in gauze in order to put more pressure on the incision. I felt like I had gone backwards, and that was really depressing.

This was also the day that the surgeon wanted us to meet with the oncologist that he had decided to refer me to. He explained that the oncologist would manage my case after I had healed from the surgery. He told us that this doctor, whose office was also in Los Angeles, was one of the top people in her field. Once again, we felt extremely fortunate that I would be treated by such a well-respected physician.

From the beginning, we were impressed with this very personable oncologist. She wanted to examine me that first day, but since I was all bandaged up, it wasn't possible. The oncologist's job was to go over the results of the tissue and lymph node tests and recommend a course of treatment. Upon meeting her, the first words out of my mouth were "Do I have to go through chemotherapy, because if there is something else, I would prefer it." I had heard all sorts of stories about people becoming deathly ill from the side effects of chemotherapy and I didn't want to go there if I didn't need to. At the time, I had hair down to the middle of my back and I did not want to lose it. Obviously, my priorities were a bit skewed. The doctor told me that some people actually beg her to put them on chemotherapy so they would have better odds, but that she didn't think it would be necessary for me. (Today there is actually a genetic test called OncotypeDX that can be done for breast cancer patients to find out if chemotherapy would be recommended or not after surgery and radiation). Her preferred treatment would be radiation at the site of the tumor (which could be done in Santa Barbara) followed by the hormone tamoxifen (Nolvodex®), which was a much heralded treatment at the time.

Tamoxifen is given to block estrogen receptors in the body—it is considered an anti-estrogen. Today, research has shown that other drugs, called aromatase inhibitors, are preferable to tamoxifen. The three aromatase inhibitors that are approved by the U.S. Food and Drug Administration are: Arimidex® (chemical name anastrazole), Femara® (chemical name letrozole) and Aromasin® (chemical name exemestane). At the time I was put on tamoxifen, it was expected that a patient would be on it for five years.

Recent research has shown that if a patient is put on tamoxifen for two and a half years, and then on an aromatase inhibitor for another two and a half years, they are one-third less likely to suffer a recurrence of their cancer than if they had taken tamoxifen the whole time. Other studies suggest tamoxifen for five years and then an aromatase inhibitor for another five years. A study that was released in 2004 at the San Antonio, Texas Breast Cancer Symposium stated that Arimidex reduced the risk of breast cancer recurring anywhere in the body by an additional 26% over and above the 50% reduction provided by tamoxifen. This data coincides with the announcement of new guidelines from the American Society of Clinical Oncology (ASCO). They recommended that for postmenopausal women whose tumors are driven by estrogen, optimal hormonal therapy should include an aromatase inhibitor as initial therapy, or after treatment with tamoxifen, in order to reduce risk of recurrence. The problem is that these new studies have left doctors and patients with an unclear path. Should a patient start taking an aromatase inhibitor immediately, take tamoxifen for two or three years first and then switch or take tamoxifen first for five years? Again, the jury is still out. I know some women who have chosen not to take tamoxifen at all, because of the toxicity of the drug and the risk of uterine cancer. This is something worth discussing with your oncologist.

My oncologist told me that my tumor was rather large and actually bordered on being classified as stage two. But, since the tissue samples and eight lymph nodes were clear of cancer, the oncologist said that it should be considered stage one breast cancer and that chemotherapy was not necessary. She also told my husband and me that tests had shown that the tumor was estrogen sensitive. We asked if this meant that estrogen in my system had caused the tumor to grow. After all, she was giving me tamoxifen to block estrogen receptors. Her answer to the question was that medical science really didn't know to an absolute certainty that estrogen caused breast cancer, so she really couldn't say whether or not that was the case. She explained that the only thing that was scientifically certain was that the tumor in some way bonded with and reacted to estrogen. We were left to form our own conclusions from this information. It was as if an 8,000-pound elephant had just come into the room, but its presence could not be proven as a scientific certainty. In the absence of scientific certainty, the doctor considered it best to pretend that the elephant just wasn't there at all. I found out several years later that estrogen definitely played a role in the development of my cancer.

The oncologist said I would need to see her in Los Angeles every three to four months for a simple blood test to monitor the tamoxifen.

As I mentioned previously, I was told that one stayed on tamoxifen for five years and if there was no recurrence of the cancer, one was considered cured. And that, it seemed, would be that. I would have a short period of radiation treatments, a trip to Los Angeles for blood tests and a five-minute meeting with the doctor every three or four months. Then, in a few years, the whole thing would be a bad memory. I clung to this prognosis.

Unfortunately, things didn't work out that way. In fact, there may have been a very different outcome if I had been aware then of some of the things that I now know only too well. First, I would have been a good bit more suspicious than my oncologist was of an extremely large, stage one tumor when only half of the recommended number of lymph nodes had been tested. Second, I would have insisted that the blood tests my oncologist administered every three to four months include a test for something called tumor markers. Tumor markers are naturally occurring proteins that are present in everyone's blood. When people have active cancer in their system, the levels of different individual proteins become elevated. In the case of breast cancer, it is a protein called CA15-3 (some oncologists test for CA 27.29 instead, which is very similar). The relation between the levels of these proteins and the activity of cancer is not a completely accurate thing. There can be false positives, and for that reason, some doctors don't believe in monitoring tumor markers. Still, they provide a quick and easy way to get an indication of the activity of cancer in a person's system. The normal range for CA15-3 at the lab I went to was 0 to 31.3 (this varies from lab to lab). Over the two years that I saw the oncologist in Los Angeles, to my knowledge, she never checked the level of CA15-3 in my blood. The first time I know of that my tumor markers were tested was after a CT scan had shown the cancer had metastasized in my liver. At that time, my level of CA15-3 was 848—more than 27 times higher than normal.

False positives aside, if my Los Angeles oncologist had routinely checked tumor markers I would have known much sooner that my cancer had spread, and probably would have been able to deal with it at a less advanced stage.

When I think back about that period, I realize that we had put all of our trust in this highly recommended oncologist. She told us that I would be fine and this was exactly what we wanted to hear. As with the surgeon, we felt like we were in good hands and that, since she was the expert, everything necessary was being done. At this time, the oncologist also wanted me to have a bone density test to be used as a base line, and to go on fosamax, a bone-strengthening drug, since my mother had had osteoporosis. I was also told to stop taking the hormone replacement tablets that had been prescribed by my gynecologist in Tucson.

As part of the treatment plan, I was to have between six and seven weeks of radiation therapy at the site of the tumor. These treatments were to be done in Santa Barbara, since I could not be expected to drive to Los Angeles five days a week for six weeks. In a directory of California physicians she found a radiation oncologist at the Cancer Center in Santa Barbara that she knew from her days at UCLA. She told me to set up an appointment with him so that I could go over everything necessary for the radiation therapy to begin.

When the surgeon felt I had healed sufficiently from the surgery, I made an appointment with the radiation oncologist. Michael went with me for the first meeting with him. It was really wonderful that he wanted to be a part of everything I was going through. We had only been married for two years and this brought us even closer together. From the first appointment, I was impressed with the Cancer Center of Santa Barbara. Everyone on the staff was pleasant and eager to help in any way they could. They had a great support team to help with questions, such as what ointment to use when you got burned by the radiation.

During my first appointment at the Cancer Center they applied tattoos to mark where on my breast the radiation beams needed to hit. I wasn't prepared for this, although I had probably been told that they would need to do some type of markings. I just hadn't realized that markings meant permanent tattoos would be applied. Other cancer patients I have spoken with were also unaware that permanent tattoos were going to be applied, until they showed up for their first appointment.

I remember lying on the cold table with tears streaming down the sides of my face. I just said the Serenity Prayer over and over. "God, grant me the serenity to accept the things I cannot change, the courage to change the things I can and the wisdom to know the difference." I needed to remind myself that I had no control over having cancer, and that I needed to be aware of what I actually did have control over. As I look back, I did let go of the things I could not change, but I did not become proactive in my treatments and precipitate change where I could. Patients can be aware of what tests they should ask for when diagnosed with cancer, and make themselves knowledgeable about what things might indicate that the cancer is spreading. Knowledge is power.

The Cancer Center was good at working out a daily schedule for radiation therapy that worked for each patient. For me it was to come in for radiation treatments the first thing each morning. I got to my office between 7:30 and 8:00 am and then left for my radiation appointment around 8:30 am. It only took a total of about 15 minutes with the undressing, radiation treatment, putting on some ointment and a pad, and then getting dressed again. I was usually back at my office by 9:30 am. I had a total of 33 treatments. The first 28 were the standard treatment of 50.4 gray to the breast. This was followed with five additional treatments at a higher intensity of 60.4 gray per session (this was called a boost) to just the upper breast area where the tumor had been removed. Fortunately for me, I didn't have any fatigue, which is a common side effect for patients going through radiation. The Cancer Center wanted me to speak with an on-staff social worker. I said I really didn't need to, that I was just fine. They insisted, so I met with her and told her all was okay. I never had to meet with her again. I think, in some ways, I felt that if I didn't talk about my cancer, it really wasn't there.

I wasn't ready at that time to deal with the emotional aspects of the disease. A good example of this was when volunteers brought beautiful potted daffodils into the Cancer Center for each of the patients going through radiation. We were told to take one of the plants home. I left mine there because I felt that it should go to someone who "really had cancer." Talk about denial! I felt that since I had been diagnosed as stage one, and did not have to go through chemotherapy, that I was cancer free. I also believed the radiation therapy and tamoxifen would prevent any further cancer from occurring. To me, all the cancer in my body had been removed along with the lump in my breast. I thought I was lucky and that my cancer had not spread, so I just let go of the worry. Ignorance is bliss. I did not take the cancer seriously enough, and that was a mistake.

I soon noticed that one unfortunate side effect of tamoxifen was weight gain. After just a few months, I had gained 15 pounds on top of the ten pounds I had gained after my surgery. I was a vegetarian, didn't drink, and ate sensibly. So why was I gaining all this weight? I am five feet three inches tall, and have always been around 120 pounds, so this was a lot of additional weight to have to deal with. As directed, I had been seeing the oncologist in Los Angeles every four months. I asked her what I could do about the weight gain. Her solution was to offer me a prescription for diet pills. I tried them for one day and couldn't sleep because they made me feel so wired. I threw them away, tried more exercise, and ate next to nothing. People kept telling me it was a blessing that I gained rather than lost weight, as so many people with cancer do. That was not comforting to me. My oncologist in Los Angeles never thought about doing a blood panel to see what my thyroid activity was. A few years later, when a more enlightened doctor checked my thyroid efficiency, he found that it was severely out of balance. I could have starved myself and still would not have lost weight. I needed to get my thyroid working properly before the weight would come off.

Shortly after I had finished my six weeks of radiation treatments, I saw a story in our local newspaper about a new 60 mile walk from Santa Barbara to Malibu to raise funds for breast cancer research. It was called the Avon 3-Day Walk. I was an avid walker, so I immediately called but found that registration had already been closed because they had reached the maximum number of walkers for that year. I made a mental note to try it the following year. It is interesting that I wanted to do this walk, since I generally didn't let anyone know that I was a breast cancer survivor. I think many people keep their cancer a secret. If that is the only way they can deal with it, that's fine. But, when I finally did start to talk about having cancer, I started to heal emotionally.

It turned out to be another two years before I would actually go on my first Avon 3-Day Walk. Little did I know that a chance meeting that year with another walker would lead me to a new and unexpected course of treatment that would change my life completely.

In the meantime, everything continued as before. My bout with cancer became a footnote, brought to mind only by the brief visits with the oncologist in Los Angeles every four months. A year and a half after the radiation and surgery were over, Michael and I went to Prague in the Czech Republic to visit my daughter, Kim. She was living there for a year and teaching English as a Second Language in a private school. My twin sister Cheryl and her husband Len joined us and we had the time of our lives—what an incredible city. While there, we saw so many Longhaired Dachshunds that I started thinking how nice it would be to get one. Michael and I have always been dog people, and at that time we had a huge and loveable Rottweiler and a very sweet black Labrador Retriever. But, I started thinking that one day we might want a smaller dog. I felt so alive and free in Prague. I never ever thought about the cancer. To me it was already a part of my past.

A month after we got back, in October 1999, I went to a Greeting Card Association Convention in Florida. It was during this convention that, for the first time, I started having a sharp pain on my right side. When I got back to Santa Barbara, Michael said he thought I must have contracted some virus in Florida. The pain got worse, but all of Michael's family and my son, Michael, were coming for Thanksgiving, so I put off going to the doctor. The people at my office noticed that I held my right side, and that I had a sore lower back. They thought that it could be a kidney infection. They told me that cranberry juice might help. I ran out to the store and bought some. It actually did seem to lessen the pain, so I drank more!

But the pain did not go away and, since it was time for my regular four-month visit to the oncologist in Los Angeles, I arranged for an appointment the Monday after Thanksgiving. My oncologist did a blood test that showed the enzyme levels in my liver were elevated. She told me to go off tamoxifen and come back for a repeat blood test the following week. She said she was concerned that I might have contracted viral hepatitis. She never mentioned the possibility that the cancer might have spread. I went back the next week and had another blood test. The enzymes were still elevated, and this time she said that I should have a CT scan, which her office arranged for me to get done in Santa Barbara the next afternoon—November 30, 1999. I'm sure most people would have started worrying about their cancer having spread. But I had become convinced the cancer was gone, and was more worried about something like hepatitis. This was all a part of my denial regarding the cancer.

The next morning, I stopped by the lab where the scan would be done and picked up the Barium oral contrast that I needed to start taking four hours before the scan. I was told that I would also have an injection of iodine contrast through a vein while the scan was in progress.

Intravenous contrast allows the physicians to examine the vascular system associated with various organs and anatomical structures. I was to have a CT scan of the chest, abdomen and pelvis. Because my veins were good, the injection was painless. The contrast made me feel very warm inside, from the throat on down.

I remember in particular that after the scan was completed, the technician was very worried that I had not listed a Santa Barbara doctor for the results to be sent to. I must have told her three times that they needed to call or fax my oncologist in Los Angeles with the results, and that she would be the one to call me. The technician was so insistent that I finally told her she could also send the results to the radiation oncologist I had seen at the Cancer Center of Santa Barbara. She was very relieved and said he would have the results that afternoon, and that a report would be faxed to my Los Angeles doctor as well. Naturally, from the technician's reaction I figured that something serious must have shown up on the scan. I don't know why, but it never even occurred to me to call the Cancer Center and speak to the radiation oncologist I had seen there to get the test results.

After the scan, I went back to my office in hopes that my oncologist would call from Los Angeles with the results. After a while, I left and went over to Michael's office to let him know that I still hadn't heard from the doctor. As I mentioned already, the doctor had called him with the bad news. When I saw him, he looked very solemn. He told me he had spoken with the doctor, and took me into his conference room to discuss what she had said. I just walked past his employees wondering what he was going to say—like I didn't already know!

After Michael related everything he'd been told, he held me close and cried. Then we called the oncologist. She said that I needed to start chemotherapy immediately or I would die, and that she would no longer be able to treat me. I would need a doctor closer to home, and she would refer me to an oncologist in Santa Barbara. That was unsettling because I had developed a rapport with her. Now I was facing a tough road, and it was going to have to be with someone totally new.

The next difficult task was calling my family and letting them know that the cancer had spread throughout my liver. How do you tell the people you love that you only have a three percent chance of beating this disease? I tried to put a positive spin on the results. I had been told that I was considered a "chemo virgin" since I did not go through chemotherapy when I first got cancer. This meant there was a better chance the chemotherapy would be effective. For me, it has always been important to know all of the facts. My philosophy is "what is, is" and worrying about the consequences won't change the facts. I also think family members need to know what's going on so they can prepare themselves to deal with it.

The first call I made was to my twin sister, and I can't really put into words how difficult that call was for me to make. But her positive attitude came through and it made the rest of the calls much easier. When I think back to the whole episode in Michael's conference room, it's a real blur. I doubt we got much sleep that night in anticipation of what was to come.

"A sure way for one to lift himself up is by helping to lift someone else."

— BOOKER T. WASHINGTON

CHAPTER TWO

Starting Chemotherapy

On December 3, 1999 I met my new oncologist, Dr. Thomas Woliver, for the first time. His office was at the Cancer Center of Santa Barbara. Before our meeting, he had reviewed the film from my CT scan and later told us that he was shocked to see me walking into his office looking so healthy. He said he had expected me to be very ill and that I might have had to be carried into his office.

I liked him immediately, and felt that I could trust him to tell me the truth about what was happening and what we needed to do. I think it is so important to feel comfortable with your doctor. If you don't, you should go to someone else. You have to trust that your questions will be truthfully answered. I think it is vital to have confidence that your doctors know what they are doing, and that they are open to new and complementary therapies. I have met several cancer patients whose doctors told them if they seek complementary therapies, they would be dropped as patients. I have a great deal of sympathy for them. Fortunately for me, my oncologist does not feel this way.

While Michael and I were in his office at that first appointment, Dr. Woliver showed us the film from my CT scan. That was when I saw the cancerous tumors for the first time. According to the written report from the radiologist, the tumors in my liver were too numerous to count and ranged in size from one to four centimeters. The scan also showed a lesion in my spleen, which they believed was a non-malignant cyst. Additionally, there was a spot on one of my vertebrae that they did not believe was malignant, but was something to monitor in the future.

While explaining all of this, Dr. Woliver came across as a very intelligent and caring physician. I felt I was in good hands. When I was in another room, dressing after my exam, Michael told him that my previous doctor said I might live for four years. Dr. Woliver said that was extremely optimistic, but that he really did not believe in giving time frames. After I had returned to the consultation room, I asked, "Have you ever treated successfully anyone with cancer worse than mine?" He said that he had, and that was all I needed to hear.

He told us that I was scheduled for a brain scan the next morning in order to see if the cancer had spread to my brain. On Monday I would have a bone scan, followed by a liver biopsy on Tuesday. My sister Cheryl and her husband Len flew over to be with me for the tests. I know all of this was especially difficult for Len because his mother had died from breast cancer and his father had died from lung cancer. Cheryl and Len have been married since college and I had lived with his parents for a few months during college. Len is like a real brother to me and is very supportive of the closeness that Cheryl and I share. Many spouses of twins find that difficult to handle, but both Cheryl and I were lucky enough to marry people who enjoy the bond we have.

An MRI (magnetic resonance imaging) is the diagnostic test of choice for detecting cancer in the brain. Mine was scheduled for Saturday morning, and we all went over for the test. I was fortunate to have so many people there to support me. I had never had an MRI before. During the test, electromagnetic energy produces detailed computer images of the brain from different angles. The MRI scanner is a tube surrounded by a giant circular magnet. I was placed on a moveable bed, which was inserted into the magnet. I was told it was important to stay still and breathe normally for the best accuracy. Loud, repetitive clicking noises can be heard as the scanning proceeds. Outside of that very loud noise, the test is painless.

I had been worried about finding that the cancer had spread to my brain, but I also remember taking comfort from just having read Lance Armstrong's autobiography. He was cancer free after his cancer had spread to his brain, so I knew that cancer that has metastasized in the brain could be treated. Knowing this helped me to relax and not panic while we waited for the results. Dr. Woliver called me at home that afternoon and told me that the scan was negative; there was no cancer in the brain. What a relief—this was the first good news we had received in what seemed like a very long time. I was surprised that a doctor would call on a Saturday afternoon to let me know the results, but I think he knew we needed some positive news.

Monday arrived and it was time for the bone scan. A bone scan, unlike the MRI, involved two steps. First I had to go in three hours before the actual scan for an injection of a small amount of a radioactive substance called radionuclide. It travels through the blood and collects in the bones. I returned three hours later and was placed on a table, and a head-to-toe scan was performed with a device called a gamma camera. The actual scan took about an hour. Later that day, Dr. Woliver again called with good news—no cancer was detected.

Next on the agenda was a liver biopsy. It was scheduled for Tuesday morning at Santa Barbara Cottage Hospital. The purpose of the test was to obtain tissue samples from the tumors in my liver. These samples would then be tested to confirm that the cancer in my liver was a metastasis of the original breast cancer, and to determine if I would be a candidate for a chemotherapy drug called Herceptin. A liver biopsy is a fairly delicate procedure. Since there is a danger that the lung or gall bladder could be damaged, the doctor performing the test has to have some way of knowing exactly where he is placing the special needle that is used to extract the tissue. In my case, the test was guided by a CT scan, and the entire procedure was performed at the CT scanner.

After they numbed me with a local anesthetic, a needle was inserted into my liver. It was totally painless. During the test, I was able to watch the monitor as the doctor did the biopsy. I realized then, for the first time, that the diagnosis really was correct—my liver was truly full of cancer. The tumors were right there in front of me on the screen! I guess you always want to think that there's some small chance someone else's scan got mixed up with yours, but here was absolute confirmation that this wasn't the case.

During the test, they had had to use a larger needle than expected, so I had to stay in a room in the hospital for four hours so I could be monitored for internal bleeding. Cheryl and Len had to leave to fly back to Tucson, so Michael just sat in a chair and kept me company. How lucky I am to have such a caring and loving husband. Finally, they let me leave and we went home. Later we found out that I was not a candidate for Herceptin. The tumors were what they called HER2/NEU-negative.

The testing continued. The next morning I had to have a MUGA (Multiple Gated Acquisition) scan. This is a non-invasive test that produces a moving image of the heart so the doctor can evaluate its pumping ability. One of the chemotherapy drugs they wanted to give me— Adriamycin—can be toxic to the heart muscle and can lead to heart failure. For the test, a small amount of blood was drawn from my arm and mixed with an imaging agent. The blood was then reinjected into my blood stream a couple of hours later. Next I had to lay on a table under the gamma camera. It acquired data based on the tagged red blood cells and my heart rate. From this data, a computer calculated the blood volume pumped through the left ventricle of my heart. The test showed that I had a strong heart, and my first chemotherapy session was scheduled for the following day.

I met with a chemotherapy nurse right after the MUGA scan, and she explained all of the side effects of the chemotherapy I would be receiving. She told me I would lose all my hair. Some chemos do not cause hair loss, but Adriamycin and Taxotere, both of which I was scheduled to have, do. She said my hair would start to fall out about three weeks after the first chemotherapy session. I was told other side effects could include nausea, fatigue, low white blood count, mouth sores, and loss of eyelashes and eyebrows. Well, I just listened and made up my mind that what would be, would be. I would get through it. I worried most about the nausea, since many medications I had taken in the past had made me throw up. I was afraid the nausea would be debilitating, but the chemo nurse explained that medicines developed to help treat AIDS patients had made nausea very manageable. That was great news to me!

As my chemotherapy was about to begin, I discovered that a great many people—who mean well and have the best of intentions—want you to know what treatments they think you should pursue. For the most part, this advice is totally unsolicited. Almost every cancer patient I have spoken with has experienced similar "good intentions" by friends, family and acquaintances. One instance that I remember only too well was when a friend of ours called to ask if I wanted a second opinion. He happens to be a physician and he called as soon as he heard about my cancer having spread. I told him that I didn't need to consult anyone else because I already had two oncologists, and that I felt confident in the people who were advising me.

In spite of my response, he proceeded to tell me that if I would get some progesterone cream, available at any health food store, and rub it on my body, the cancer would go away. This was amazing to me, and sounded so completely bizarre. It was especially unsettling because he is a physician. After I told this story to my Los Angeles oncologist, she said, "Carol, progesterone cream will not cure your cancer." Believe me, I already knew that. It might have actually been harmful to me, as I later learned that I had an overabundance of progesterone in my body. At that time, however, I was under a great deal of stress, felt emotionally fragile, and just did not need this unsolicited advice.

Many years later I read that progesterone cream is something some doctors prescribe for lumpy, painful breasts. I have not heard it will cure cancer that has metastasized in the liver. I have also learned that before taking anything like progesterone or estrogen, you need to find out what the levels of these hormones are in your body. Too much estrogen or progesterone can be dangerous. Many caring people want to hand out free advice, and it is important to remember that they mean well. But, some advice can be harmful. I have heard stories from doctors and nurses of people who have been lured to supposed miracle treatments, and then put off chemotherapy until it is too late.

It is important to be extremely careful and diligent in your research before foregoing traditional treatments for untested alternatives. I am not saying to avoid complementary treatments. To the contrary, I think it is extremely important to pursue them. But, in my case, as you will learn, I did it in conjunction with conventional medicines. It's hard for cancer patients to sift through all the advice that will be freely given, but checking out hospitals and medical schools in the United States that have departments for alternative or complementary medicine is a good start. Other cancer patients can also be good sources of information.

I thoroughly checked out the complementary treatments that I ended up pursuing, and discussed them with my oncologist to get his opinion. It is important to be aware that each of our bodies is different, and that a therapy good for one person may not be good for another. Learning as much as possible about your own body is imperative. For example, I have read books giving blanket advice that soy is good for you. Yet, I know for a fact that I need to avoid soy, because my body has too much estrogen (something I learned a few years later in a simple blood test), and soy contains estrogen.

My first chemotherapy session took place on December 10, 1999. Dr. Woliver had told us he wanted to get in six cycles of chemotherapy scheduled three weeks apart. I went in feeling fairly well-prepared and knowing what to expect. The chemo nurses were very friendly and tried to explain each of the different bags that went up on the I.V. stand. I was fortunate in that my veins were not hard to find. I'm not saying it didn't hurt when I was stuck, but the pain was over quickly.

I've read stories about patients looking at the fluids going into their veins and feeling overwhelmed by the thought of the toxicity of the drugs. I have to admit, that never occurred to me. I had read about the "red poison" called Adriamycin that was being put into my body, but at the time I was actually hoping it would be toxic enough to kill the cancer. I felt that my body was very strong and that I would be able to handle the chemotherapy. I now understand what other people were feeling and why they were fearful of these toxic drugs. I believe those patients had a healthy fear. At that time, I was merely in survival mode. I knew that time was not on my side and I needed to do everything I could to extend the time I had.

I had been given a prescription for Decadron tablets and was told to start taking them before the first chemotherapy session. Decadron is a steroid used to prevent nausea and vomiting for patients going through chemotherapy. In the past, cancer patients did not have access to such incredible drugs to help with these side effects.

Before being given Adriamycin and Taxotere (the big guns, as they were called), I first received an intravenous combination of Anzemet (to prevent nausea) and Decadron (to prevent nausea, decrease the fluid retentive effects of Taxotere, and to improve my sense of 'well-being'). I'm sure this is why I really didn't have problems with nausea. I was also given a prescription for Compazine and Ativan, which are anti-nausea medicines that are modestly tranquilizing on their own.

A couple of days after the chemo I felt some gastric discomfort, but Compazine did the trick. I was able to not only handle the chemotherapy, but go on with my normal activities. I can't stress enough how much this meant to me. Being able to go on with my life as though the chemo was just part of the normal routine helped me to cope. That was how I had looked at going through radiation two years earlier. Taking off work and staying home sick was not for me. My side effects were very manageable. Some patients are not so fortunate and they can't resume their normal activities. But most cancer patients I have met were able to handle chemotherapy without too much difficulty. When I had trouble sleeping, because I was worrying about having cancer and being able to still run my company, Ativan helped to settle me down. When I found out that Ativan could be addictive, I only used it when I really had problems getting to sleep.

Probably, running my company helped me to focus on something other than the cancer. I really didn't have any choice in the matter. When you own a small business, you can't just have someone else take over. I had the responsibility of making a weekly payroll, paying the bills, and deciding on the artwork for new greeting cards we would be introducing. I did turn over attending trade shows to my director of marketing, since I had to worry about avoiding crowds when my white count was low. Nevertheless, along with owning the company came a great deal of stress—which was not good for fighting cancer.

After my first chemotherapy session, I decided to find a wig before my hair started to fall out. I asked at the Cancer Center and they gave me a number of someone who could help. She came to the Cancer Center once a week from Los Angeles, where she had a shop. Michael and I decided to go to her shop, thinking that there would be more wigs to choose from. She was very nice and helped us find a wig and some hats. I had heard that with a bald head I would get cold at night when I took my wig off to go to bed. I soon learned they were right about that! Just having the wig made me feel more prepared for when my hair would start to come out. It was like a security blanket. I clung to whatever made me feel I could handle the situation I had been presented with. Many choose to wear scarves and some people look great in them, but I wasn't one of them. At the time, I also did not want to "look" like I was in chemotherapy. I had a company to run and I didn't want people thinking I wouldn't be able to handle the things going on at work. Now that I look back, it was ridiculous to feel that way, but that's how things were at the time. I didn't want to be treated any differently than before I had cancer. I'm sure this was how I was able to handle everything that was going on. Some people can't stand to wear a wig and have all sorts of scarves and hats. Maybe if I lose my hair again I will go that route!

I made an appointment to get my hair cut off. I had heard horror stories of people's hair falling out in the shower, and I didn't think I could bear to have that happen. The vision of my long strands coming out in my hand was hard to imagine. I had had long hair for the last 20 years, and it was one thing that helped people distinguish me from my twin sister. This was going to be quite a change for me.

My hairdresser was very upset at the prospect of having to cut my hair. I think she found it difficult to accept the fact that my cancer had spread. Her own father was dealing with cancer at the time and he wasn't doing well. At first, she cut my hair to just about chin length. I called her a few days later and told her I wanted to come back and have it cut really short. I could just feel her discomfort when I came back in for the next appointment. She had taken care of my hair for many years and knew how much I liked it long. I had always dreamed about growing old with a long braid twisted on top of my head, like my great-grandmother. I had also felt that Katherine Hepburn grew old very graciously, with her hair piled up on top of her head. I wanted to be like her. While I knew intellectually that hair would grow back, my fear was that it would grow back and then I would have to go through chemotherapy again and lose it all a second time. I knew the cancer was in my lymph system and that it could show up in another part of my body at any time. The fact that my hairdresser was nervous around me made me realize that cancer affects everyone you are associated with. Some people have such a great fear of cancer that they don't know how to react around someone who has it. Maybe they feel vulnerable.

After getting my hair cut I decided that it was time to call my banker and set up a lunch meeting. I knew I needed to tell her about the cancer. I wanted to explain everything, let her see that I was okay, and reassure her that there would be no problem paying back my line of credit. Having a line of credit is important in the greeting card business because of its seasonal nature. Each year a new holiday catalog had to be prepared for the trade shows in May. Stores wanted their holiday card orders shipped in August. That meant we had to go to press in June and hire extra staff to start putting the orders together. But we wouldn't get paid for those orders until September at the earliest and, in many cases, not until December or January.

My banker was pretty straightforward. She wanted to know the prognosis. I reminded her that my line of credit was secured with a life insurance policy for more than I owed. I knew that she needed to ask those questions. That was her job and I expected her to do it. She had always been there for my company, treating me with as much respect as her much larger clients. She actually ended up becoming the CEO and President of that bank, and I still consider her a dear friend.

About eight days after my first chemotherapy session, my white cell count plummeted and I had to go in for daily shots of a drug called Neupogen to bring my white count up. It was not a comfortable shot, and I had to have it for three days in a row that first time. Some nurses were better than others, and would try to warm the vial containing the drug in their hands before giving the injection. That did help. Perhaps, for some patients, it is no big deal, but I happen to hate shots. Naturally, I got accustomed to them. Today there is a new slow-release version of Neupogen called Neulasta. It is equivalent to 12 days of Neupogen and costs as much! Few patients need 12 days however, much less the $6,000 retail price tag. Although, for me, it would have been preferable to have one injection instead of daily shots for three to five days in a row. When they tell you that you have to come in daily for the injections, it means every day—including Saturday and Sunday. You also had to have regular blood tests to see if the white count is going up. Because the Cancer Center was closed on the weekends, the doctors would come in and take turns giving the shots themselves. I got to know all of the oncologists at the Cancer Center that way, and found out who was better at giving injections. I personally thought Dr. Woliver was the best!

Michael and I felt we needed to get away from all of the medical stuff, and since our fourth wedding anniversary was coming up, we decided to go to Disneyland. It was just a short drive away and my white count was normal, so I didn't have to worry about being around people. We would return the day before I would have to start my second chemotherapy session. It had been almost three weeks since my first chemo and my hair was falling out, so I brought my wig and hats to Disneyland. I remember holding on tight to my hat during the rides fearing that it would fly off with the wig and land on some unsuspecting child, scaring them!

It was fun to be in a totally different environment, but we both had a lot on our minds—so much had happened in such a short time. It had only been one month since the diagnosis. Our lives had changed so drastically and would never be the same again. Our vocabulary would now include such words as chemotherapy, neupogen, compazine, ativan, tumor markers, lymph nodes—everything that went along with having fourth-stage breast cancer. I was fighting a life-threatening disease and we both knew that every day was precious. There was no turning back the clock. This was what we were going to have to face from now on. I had no choice in the matter, but those around me had to have a lot of courage to stick it out and watch someone they love go through all of this.

As we were celebrating our four years together, I did a lot of thinking about how Michael and I had met. At the time of our meeting, I had been very involved in mentoring young women in jail. I would help get them into treatment for alcohol and drug abuse. I had been molested as a child and knew that a high percentage of the women in jail had also been sexually abused. Since I had been able to get beyond the trauma of my youth, go to college and graduate school, and start my own business; I had been told I could be a role model for these women. My twin sister became a psychologist and worked with women and children who had been abused. She gave them the help I never had. Her work had a big influence on me—I wanted to do something that could make a difference in someone's life. I had always done volunteer work and felt strongly that people should extend themselves beyond their job.

Still, I questioned how these women would feel about me, since I had never been in jail. I was afraid they would think I was "full of it"—not really understanding where they were coming from. The director of the program told me that these women didn't need to learn more about being in jail, they needed to learn how to succeed in life outside of jail. That sounded convincing to me, so I signed up.

Through my work at the jail, I came across a girl I will call Robin, whose drug use had gotten her into trouble several times. She was very bright and from a good family, but when I first met her I knew she was not ready to get help. She was still excited about the life she was living as a heroin addict. She got out of jail and then, a few months later, I saw her back in jail. She had hit rock bottom. She was 23 years old and was awaiting trial for possession of narcotics. The charges were all the more serious because she had violated the terms of her probation from an earlier charge, as well as the terms of her parole from a previous conviction.

Robin asked me to work with her one-on-one. I said I would only do it if I felt she was serious about addressing her problems. She convinced me that she was, and promised she would do whatever I asked. I told her this would be a lifetime commitment on my part and that I would be there for her as long as she was willing to work on her problems. This blew her away—no one had ever said that to her. One of my requirements was that she call me every day from jail on my company's toll free line. This she did. I also asked her to write down everything about how her addiction had impacted her life and that we would go over it in detail. I don't know how to explain what I felt, but somehow I connected with Robin from the first time I saw her.

When I met with the girls at the jail in a group, it was in one of the cells or one of the education rooms. I was right with them. But if I was meeting with just one of them, it had to be in a small cubicle with a glass wall between us and a headset to speak through. When Robin and I met, we tried to get the room that had a place to slide papers through the glass wall—this was the one where lawyers met with their clients. That way I could have Robin work on writing things down and then I could read them. I could see by the way she expressed herself in writing that she was very bright. She had left high school before graduating, but I could see she had a tremendous amount of potential. I had taught Social Documentary Photography and Photojournalism at the University of Arizona and had read many college papers. These papers, written in jail by a high school dropout, were better than some of the ones that had been written by former college students of mine! I knew that Robin had the ability to not only get her GED, but to go on to college.

At one point I asked Robin if she had been sexually abused as a child. She wondered how I knew that she had been, and I told her about my own experience. I also told her I felt she might be using drugs to forget the abuse. She told me about the abuse, which had been at the hands of a family friend when she was very young. Many years earlier, she had to testify in court against him. At the time she felt very conflicted, because he had been a friend of the family and had told her that what went on between them was their secret. By testifying in court, she was violating this secret. In the intervening years, this had become a huge emotional issue for her and drugs had become her escape. She told me that she had never confided to anyone about the abuse—she just tried to block it from her memory. After an extremely troubled adolescence, she had been on the streets since 16, hooked on heroin by 18, and had had eight serious overdoses—including two which generated calls to 911 saying that she was dead.

I called my twin sister and asked her for a referral to a good residential treatment program for Robin. She told me about one in New England, near the town that her parents had moved to from Santa Barbara. Robin wanted to be closer to her mother. I called the treatment center and found that they would also be able to arrange therapy for Robin for the abuse issue. I then arranged a telephone interview between the treatment center and Robin. She was accepted, if the courts would allow her to go there. I knew her parents had enough money to pay for the program, so fortunately that would not be a problem. The next step was to get the assistant district attorney assigned to her case to accept this program instead of sending Robin to prison. We were lucky to have a caring assistant district attorney on her case. She knew all about Robin's problems over the years, but had never heard about the abuse during her childhood. She told me that she always felt something was wrong with Robin, since it appeared that she was trying to kill herself. Robin had overdosed the last time she was arrested, and the DA told me she overheard policemen betting each other that the next time they saw her, she would be in the morgue.

The assistant district attorney invited me to present information about the residential treatment program in a private session in the judge's chambers, which her probation officer would also attend. I had a full description of the program in New England to give to the judge, the probation officer, and the district attorney. I explained it was an intensive year-long program—not one of the miracle 90-day cures they were used to hearing about. The program seemed to impress them and they agreed that Robin could go, even though the probation officer had already typed up a recommendation for a three-year prison sentence.

Of all times, I had to be in New York for the National Stationery Show when Robin's parole hearing was scheduled. This hearing was the last thing standing in the way of the treatment program. A counselor from the jail who had been working with Robin went to the hearing to speak on her behalf. Unfortunately, the parole board said they weren't about to let Robin go off to this cozy little program. They said she needed to spend a year in prison to "think" about what she had done. What a waste—I knew prison was not the answer for someone like Robin. She was not a threat to anyone but herself.

I received a call in New York from Robin, telling me what had happened. I was devastated, and worried that she would give up and start using drugs again. They were so accessible in jail. But she didn't. The moment my plane landed in Santa Barbara, I went directly to the jail to meet with her. They had a lenient policy at the Santa Barbara Jail, and I could meet with the women I was mentoring at most any time. Robin explained that she had accepted the year in prison—that I had taught her that things happen for a reason, and that she would go to AA and NA meetings in prison. We discussed how she could get her GED while in prison. She said she would write me every day. She knew that in order to keep the spot available at the treatment program in New England, she would also have to write them once a week. We both cried because we knew this would be the last visit we would have for a year. She was being transferred to prison the next morning.

Over the next year, Robin called me as often as she could and she wrote me every day. I was so impressed with the complete turn-around in her life. It wasn't easy for her to stay away from drugs in prison. They were offered to her but she told the people around her that she wanted to stay clean and they respected her wishes. She worked out at the track and took every class she could to keep herself busy. One of the things I had Robin do was to write down her goals in life. As with most of the women I worked with, this was a new concept. I explained to Robin that she had to be very clear, and come up with a set of detailed life goals. I told her that if she could do that and stay focused, she could accomplish those goals. She said this helped her to concentrate on what she really wanted to do. I explained that if she could stay clean, going to college was a very realistic goal. I told her that she was more than bright enough. This was something no one had ever said to her before, and it gave her something to work towards.

Ten months later, when she was released from prison, I was there to pick her up and bring her back to Santa Barbara. We still didn't have approval for her to leave the state for the treatment program in New England, so I got her checked into a local treatment facility until the approval came through. I knew someone at the probation office and I went to him and explained that I was totally frustrated that it was taking so long to get approval from the parole board. I told him I was worried because I could see Robin acting a little different and spending time talking to people she knew from her heroin days. She was still clean, but she needed to get away from her old environment as soon as possible. The next day the approval came through and off Robin and I flew to New England. As part of the requirements of her probation I was to travel with her to the residential treatment program.

We spent the weekend at her parents' house in New England. It was beautiful, with snow all over the place. I had lived in New York but had never been to that part of New England. It exceeded all of my expectations. When I discovered that Robin's stepfather was an artist, I suggested we might work together to create greeting cards depicting some of the images from his artwork. He said he would love to do that, and mentioned that a friend of his, named Michael Silverander, was a graphic designer in Santa Barbara. He said he would want him to work on the design of the cards.

I made an appointment with and met Michael shortly after my return to Santa Barbara. I was impressed with him at our first meeting. He came across as being extremely knowledgeable about graphic design and he was very personable. I was physically attracted to him and pleased to learn that he was single. It turned out that our offices were only a block and a half apart. The next day, on an afternoon walk with his new little Rottweiler puppy, Riley, he stopped by my office to say hello. We soon learned just how much we had in common. Santa Barbara was a small community, and since our businesses were so similar in so many ways, it was amazing we hadn't met sooner. We had both been single for many years. The timing was perfect. It didn't take long before we fell in love. We got married nine months later and our wedding was like a chapter from a romance novel. Because of my work with Robin, I met the man of my dreams. It was so wonderful to have Robin there at the wedding, to share in my happiness. She is as close to me as any member of my own family.

Robin successfully completed the residential treatment program, although it was difficult and there were times when she was ready to pack it in. After the program, she went on to college and graduated summa cum laude with a degree in business. Robin beat the odds and conquered her heroin addiction. Today, besides holding down a full-time job, she is enrolled in a program to get her MBA. We stay in close touch even though she lives on the East Coast. The strength that Robin displayed in conquering her addiction has been an inspiration to me in my battle with cancer.

"Laughter is a tranquilizer with no side effects."

—ARNOLD GLASOW

CHAPTER THREE

Cancer on My Rib and a New Puppy

Michael and I returned from celebrating our anniversary at Disneyland, and I had my second chemotherapy session the next day—New Year's Eve, December 31, 1999. Before each chemo infusion, Michael and I would meet with the oncologist. He had to confirm that I was physically up to another dose of chemotherapy. We went over my most recent blood test and at the appointment before my second chemo, I learned that my tumor markers (CA15-3) had dropped from 848 to 770.7 (normal being 31.3 and lower). I still had a long way to go to get into the normal range! I told the doctor that my eyes had been watering and found that this was a normal reaction to the chemo I had been given. Other than that, it appeared I was handling the chemotherapy without too much difficulty.

Cheryl and Len flew over from Tucson so we could celebrate the dawning of the new century at our house. Again, Compazine and Ativan proved to be a big help in keeping down the side effects of the chemotherapy. I felt bad that we couldn't go out for a nice dinner, but I just wasn't up for it. Everything still was so new. I showed Cheryl how my hair was coming out. It made my scalp sore. It was nice that Cheryl came over for the chemotherapy sessions and this time, I showed her a new wig that I had purchased. It looked more real than the first one. It was cute and it made me feel normal. I think this was especially important for me in handling the hair loss and in having cancer in general—feeling "normal." If I felt normal it was as though cancer wasn't this huge uncontrollable thing. It made everything less frightening.

Again, my white cell count went way down—actually I was told that I had "virtually no white blood cells." This time I had to have Neupogen shots for four days in a row before my white count went up. Since my immune system was compromised, getting sick or having a fever was a big concern. I was told if my fever ever got to 101 degrees, I was to immediately call the Cancer Center and get a prescription for an antibiotic. The weekend I went in for Neupogen shots I was not feeling particularly well. By the time I got home and took my temperature, it was over 102. We telephoned the oncologist on call. She ordered an antibiotic and said if the fever did not go down, we were to go directly to the hospital. By the time Michael came back with the medicine, my fever was over 103. I used cool compresses on my forehead all night long and even took a tepid bath. Michael started getting worried and wanted to take me to the hospital, but I wanted to see if the antibiotic would work. Finally the fever broke. I was so relieved not to have to go to the hospital.

I started to feel like I was getting used to the routine and to wearing the wig, but my head was getting really sore. Every time I took the wig off, there were clumps of hair stuck inside it. I decided to bite the bullet and have Michael shave my head. I am sure this was difficult for him, and I cried after seeing myself completely bald. But it was actually much better that way. Immediately, I noticed my scalp was not as sore. Still, every time I took off my hats or wig, like in the morning for a shower, I had to look at my bald head in the mirror and that was very hard. I used to cry in the shower, which was actually a great stress reliever.

Cheryl and I used to speak on the telephone frequently, but after my cancer metastasized, we spoke several times every day. This still continues. In fact, if evening comes and I haven't spoken with her it feels funny, and I call. When you are as "connected at the hip" as we are, there is always something to say. I don't know how Cheryl handles my cancer. I'm also very close to my sister Nancy, but twins are different—you feel like you are part of one another. I have spoken with other twins and this is something we all seem to have in common. My twin nieces are also extremely close to each other. I really don't know how I could watch Cheryl have a life threatening disease—I feel so badly what she has to go through every day with the thought of me possibly dying. It doesn't seem fair, because many years ago she lost a child to congenital heart disease when he was only a year old. I feel I must work hard to stay well and strong for her.

While I was going through chemotherapy, a friend of Cheryl's said that her brother had done research on the internet and found that a nutritional supplement called IP-6 (purportedly an immune enhancer) could help combat cancer. We were told that a book had been written by a pathologist, Dr. AbulKalam M. Shamsuddin, a Professor of Pathology at the University of Maryland School of Medicine in Baltimore, regarding the amazing results of taking the B-vitamin inositol and its derivative inositol hexaphosphate (IP-6). Apparently it would prevent the formation of cancer and even shrink pre-existing cancers. Several years later, I found out that the University of Maryland School of Medicine has an active department dealing with complementary medicines. This sounded interesting to Michael and me. We spoke to Dr. Woliver about my taking inositol and IP-6 and he didn't have a problem with it. He was pretty open to complementary treatments as long as he felt they didn't put my health in jeopardy.

This friend of Cheryl's had actually made up a recipe of sorts, combining various vitamins, but mostly inositol and IP-6. We bought all of the ingredients at a health food store and started opening up all of the capsules to make the concoction. We needed to open, empty, and combine the contents of more than 300 capsules for a week's supply. We were told to mix the resulting powder in a liter of apricot or peach nectar. I was to take two ounces of the mixture every morning and evening. I love apricot nectar, so that wasn't a problem. It was, however, quite time consuming. I was very diligent and took the supplement every day. I'm not sure if this helped me or not, but my energy level was never a problem throughout chemotherapy. We were willing to explore various treatments that seemed within reason.

I know people who are consumed with finding out everything they can about treatments for cancer on the internet. But it's important to remember that this can be a dangerous practice. There are a lot of good sites by trustworthy non-profit organizations like the American Cancer Society, breastcancer.org and the Susan G. Komen Foundation. They are full of valuable information. Remember, just because you find it on a web site on the internet, it's not necessarily true. Also remember that a good therapy for one person may not be good for another. Today I realize the importance of having a complete blood analysis and getting my doctor's advice before trying any new treatment.

At about this time, I told Michael I thought it might be a good idea to get a puppy. I felt it would be just the thing to take my mind off of the chemotherapy. It's not that we needed to add another dog to our family! As I mentioned, we had a 125-pound Rottweiler named Riley (who thought he was a lap dog) and a wonderful black Labrador named Katie. I just thought that a Longhaired Dachshund puppy like the ones we had seen in Prague would be therapeutic. Michael agreed and the search began. I combed the Sunday newspaper in Santa Barbara and found nothing. I called Cheryl and had her check the Tucson newspaper. Timing is everything. That Sunday, there was an ad for a brand new litter of Longhaired Dachshund puppies in the Tucson newspaper. Among the puppies, it mentioned that there was a female with a red coat and black-tipped ears. I told Cheryl to call immediately and see if she was still available. Cheryl was the first person to call in response to the ad and so we were able to get the pick of the litter. I've always thought that things that happen this perfectly are "God shots."

The breeder, Judy, was wonderful and invited Cheryl and Nancy out the next weekend to see the puppies and meet the parents of my new dog. They took lots of pictures and sent them to me. Judy even sent me a videotape of my new puppy so I could watch her grow. She was so tiny, and expressed such personality in the video that I couldn't wait until she was old enough to leave the litter and come home to be the newest member of our family. We thought about names, and "Mattie" seemed to fit her perfectly.

My third chemotherapy infusion was January 21, 2000. In the meeting with Dr. Woliver prior to the chemo, we discussed setting up another CT scan in two weeks, which would work out to be the week before my fourth chemotherapy session. Dr. Woliver was impressed that I still didn't have any fatigue. He said I would need to have another MUGA scan after the fourth session to see if my heart was strong enough to go through six cycles. With the third chemo session came another drop in my white count. I was getting very used to the Neupogen shots. They were a part of every treatment and would continue to be throughout all the remaining cycles.

After my third chemo, my daughter, Kim, came home from Prague, She was a great help by preparing meals that tasted good. Most foods had a metallic taste because of the particular chemotherapy drugs that I was on. Other chemos do not have that side effect. She made me miso soup. That was the best, along with salads. A restaurant where Michael and I frequently ate lunch had a spicy seafood gumbo on the menu that tasted great during that time. (I had added fish back to my diet for protein). The people who ran the restaurant were very understanding about my being on chemotherapy. They would seat me in a side room that was closed to everyone else during the times when my white count was low and I was susceptible to germs. This allowed me to still be able to go out for meals. Soup was especially soothing because I had sores on the inside of my mouth from the chemo. That made chewing most foods very uncomfortable.

Kim stayed in Santa Barbara for about a month and then went to San Francisco to visit friends. After that she packed up and left for Slovania, where she had another job teaching English. She didn't stay there too long. Soon, she was in Bordeaux, learning French, and then going to the Sorbonne in Paris for more classes. She lived in Paris, in a loft apartment on the Left Bank, for about a year. She learned to speak the language well and passed a difficult language proficiency exam given by the French government. I think living in different countries is so educational. Before starting my greeting card company, I had been a social documentary photographer and photojournalist. I traveled all over the world on assignments, covering events like the World Gathering of Holocaust Survivors in Israel, and going on a fact finding mission to Ethiopia. I used to go to my kids' elementary school classes and do slide shows about my trips. Maybe Kim got a little bit of the wanderlust from me.

I continued to go to work every day without experiencing problems with fatigue. I even started walking on my treadmill for about 45 minutes a day. At the urging of my son, Michael, I had purchased the treadmill when I was first diagnosed with stage one breast cancer. The idea was for me to get in shape after the surgery and radiation. I think staying in good physical shape by walking as often as possible helped with my recuperation. It's also important mentally. I think that feeling strong physically helps to develop a sense of well-being.

I wish I had been introduced to yoga at the beginning of my battle with cancer. Today, I go to yoga three times a week for strength and empowerment. I have also found yoga to be very healing. There are yoga classes for cancer patients that are offered free of charge at the Wellness Center which is part of the Cancer Center of Santa Barbara. We are lucky that the Wellness Center believes strongly in promoting activities that help cancer patients both physically and mentally. In addition to yoga, there are classes for journal writing, T'ai Chi Chih (which can stimulate the immune system), poetry, laughing for the health of it, painting, meditation, etc. Many of the patients that I have met at my yoga classes have just been diagnosed with cancer and are availing themselves of these wonderful activities. I wish I had been aware of them sooner. All these activities are very helpful in dealing with cancer. I know that many other cancer centers in other cities offer similar classes for their patients.

It was soon time for us to meet with Dr. Woliver and see the results of my most recent CT scan. A review of the film showed that the tumors appeared unchanged from the previous scan. Looking closely at the film, we all thought that there might have been more improvement than the radiologist had reported. Visually, it did appear that the largest tumors were a bit smaller. But, according to the report, they didn't measure out that way. I think we were all a bit discouraged, but the decision was made to continue on through the full six cycles of chemotherapy. At times like this, I would often go out to the deck on the back of our house and just look at the mountains behind Santa Barbara. It allowed me to reflect on everything that was going on. There is something so tranquil about watching the sun and clouds move over the mountains. I don't think I would want to live anywhere without mountains.

This was an emotional time and I couldn't help thinking about what might happen if the chemotherapy didn't work. It wouldn't be normal not to have thoughts like this and, for me, it was important to just feel the feelings. It usually didn't last long and then I would get right back into living my life.

This was when Cheryl and I both signed up to participate in the Avon 3-Day Walk to raise funds for breast cancer research. As I mentioned previously, it would turn out to be a life-altering experience. The walk took place in October and went from Santa Barbara to Malibu—a distance of 60 miles. That meant walking 20 miles per day. Cheryl and I loved to walk and we both felt that 20 miles a day was doable. I was still in chemotherapy, but knew that the walk would occur about five months after my last chemotherapy cycle. It was nice to have something to look forward to. I also loved the idea of doing this with my twin. There would be two nights in a two-person tent, and I thought it would be like a slumber party for us.

Every participant in the walk was required to raise a minimum of $1,500 in pledges. It was hard for me to write the letter asking for donations because it meant I would have to open the packet from the organizers of the walk that was filled with detailed information about cancer statistics. They felt that this information would be helpful in writing the letter. It was still too difficult for me to read those statistics. It's not that I didn't already know them only too well. It's just that it was still hard to see them in print. I ended up copying the letter that Cheryl had written and changing the name. It was the best I could do that year. Probably a more heartfelt letter about my own cancer would have been better, but talking about my cancer came later—I wasn't ready yet.

My fourth chemotherapy infusion took place on February 11, 2000. In the meeting with Dr. Woliver before the infusion, I told him I had been experiencing pain on my left side at the bottom of my rib cage. I wondered if I might have pulled a muscle while we moved some furniture the previous weekend. Dr. Woliver ordered an x-ray which didn't show anything abnormal. He said if the pain continued, we should order another bone scan just to rule out a spread of the cancer. I don't know why this didn't alarm me. I think I was still in survival mode, doing whatever needed to be done in order to deal with the cancer. So, if it was a tumor on my rib, then it would be dealt with.

My attention switched from the possibility of cancer on my rib to the fact that we were leaving the next day for Tucson to pick up our new dog, Mattie. I was so excited. We had scheduled the flight for the day after my chemotherapy. This was before my white count usually went down, which was generally eight days after chemotherapy. When we arrived in Tucson Cheryl, Len and Nancy picked us up and we all drove over to get Mattie.

This puppy was by far the cutest thing I had ever laid eyes on. I held her in my arms and she was not much bigger than my hand. We saw her parents and she looked like both of them. The rest of the litter was already gone, so we were not able to see her brothers and sisters. The breeder explained that Dachshunds like to sleep under the covers with their owners. I told her that I loved that trait. She told us that one man who had come to see the puppies said he would break his puppy of that habit. He thought dogs didn't belong on a bed. She was a good breeder, and she told this man he should go look for another breed of dog. She told him that if he tried to change the dog's disposition both he and the dog would then be miserable, and that she would not sell him one of her puppies. That night, Mattie did just what the breeder said, and snuggled right next to me under the covers. Today I am still amused watching Mattie burrow her way under the covers at night. In the morning, it is such a joy to watch her stick her head out from under the covers to lick us both in the face while her tail is going 90 miles an hour.

Before leaving Tucson, we stopped at a pet store and got a pet carrier, some puppy food and toys. Then we went back to Cheryl and Len's house where Mattie met her cousins Chrissy (Cheryl and Len's Shih Tzu) and Duffy (Nancy's Scottie). It was so funny because she ran around and was totally in their faces—no fear, even though she was a quarter of their size. This was great to see because we had wondered how she was going to handle our big dogs. I knew that Katie, our Lab, would not be a problem as she was gentle and rather timid, but Riley the Rottweiler didn't really know how big and strong he was.

The next day as we left to go back to Santa Barbara, I was really feeling nauseous. So, that was what the Compazine was for. It really helped get me through the plane ride. When we got home, we held Mattie in our arms and had the dogs sniff her out. When Riley put his mouth around her neck Mattie just sat there. Then she got right in his face and barked at him. I think he respected her spunk. It was so cute to watch their interchange. If she ever felt threatened by his size, she would scoot under the bed where he couldn't get at her. We were very lucky, Riley could have easily hurt Mattie because he was so big, but he was always extremely gentle with her.

I call Mattie my chemo dog because she played a huge role in improving my mental outlook. She still makes me laugh every single day, and that is the best medicine for anyone—especially someone fighting a disease like cancer. Mattie's participation was also a big help during all of the training walks I took to get into shape for the Avon 3-Day Walk.

By the way, Mattie curled up in a little dog bed next to my chair every day as I wrote this book. My stepson David once made a comment to his dad that while Mattie was certainly cute, the fact that we seemed to notice how cute she was at least 50 times a day was beyond him!

The pain around my lower rib continued to bother me. Dr. Woliver felt it would be best if I had a bone scan since other tests had offered no explanation for the pain. On February 28th I had a third MUGA scan to see if I could withstand the next two chemotherapy cycles (which I was cleared to do) and, the next day I had the bone scan. It seemed like the Cancer Center of Santa Barbara was my second home. Fortunately for me, it is only five minutes from my house!

It was a good thing I told the technician doing the bone scan about the pain around my rib. He decided to do an enlargement of that area, which was the only way they saw the small tumor on my ninth rib. When the radiologist first looked at the scan, he thought it was negative. Then he saw the enlargement, and there it was!

Dr. Woliver called and gave me the news. The cancer had now metastasized on my rib. I knew that since cancer travels through the lymph system, it could show up practically anywhere in my body. I was scheduled to have radiation on my rib, with 37.5 gray per treatment for five days a week for three weeks. It was hoped that that would get rid of the tumor and relieve the pain. Since I had previously had radiation on my breast at the Cancer Center, I already knew what to expect. This time I was not surprised by the tattoo. Going to the Cancer Center for radiation became a part of my daily activities for the next three weeks.

Dr. Woliver also felt that it would be good to have a PET (Positron Emission Tomography) scan to be sure that the cancer had not spread to other parts of my body. I was instructed to eat nothing after midnight the night before my scan. The next morning I was given an injection of a chemical called radionuclide combined with sugar. This is what would show up in the scan. The fact that tumors prefer sugar as an energy source is why PET scans work. It was interesting to see the results of the scan, because all of the tumors lit up, making it very obvious where the cancer was. Only the tumors on the rib and in the liver showed up in the scan. It was a relief to see that the cancer had not spread further. PET scans are very useful when trying to determine whether or not cancer has metastasized, plus they can be great for peace of mind. Some insurance companies don't cover the cost of a PET scan, which I think is unconscionable!

After the cancer was discovered on my rib, Aredia (a bone resorption inhibitor) was added to my chemotherapy regime. This was done to prevent another occurrence of cancer on the bone and to relieve the bone pain. Before the drug was prescribed for me, I remember that at one of my chemo sessions a patient sitting next to me was getting Aredia. She said it was a miracle drug for bone cancer and that she was thrilled to be getting it. You can pick up a lot of interesting information in the many hours you sit during a chemotherapy infusion. I became very flushed in the cheeks each time I received the Aredia—it was a weird feeling, but it didn't last. Adding Aredia made my chemo sessions last an additional two hours.

Today, Zometa is usually given instead of Aredia. The infusion time is also lower for Zometa—anywhere from 15 to 30 minutes. Both drugs can be nephrotoxic and kidney function must be monitored. The rate of infusion is important in both; if either is infused too rapidly, kidney dysfunction may result.

Because the chemotherapy infusions lasted so long—some more than four hours—I started reading the Harry Potter books while I was sitting there. What a great diversion for someone going through chemotherapy, it just made the time fly. I laughed so hard and was so impressed with the creativity of the entire series. I think it would be great to have the Harry Potter books available for patients to read in every cancer center. It would help adults as well as children get through their chemo sessions with a smile on their face.

In February, cancer touched my life in again in an unexpected way. Joyce, the shipping manager at my greeting card company, was diagnosed with breast cancer. I was glad that I was able to speak with her and her husband at length about what to expect and what to ask the doctors. Cancer cells had been found in 9 of the 19 lymph nodes taken during her surgery, but no other tumors were found. I was thankful that they had taken a decent number of lymph nodes in her case. When Joyce started chemotherapy I told her about the wig person I went to, and she got a great wig. She told me that watching me continue my normal activities during chemotherapy and radiation gave her confidence that she could do the same. Joyce was given Taxol and Adriamycin, she had an adverse reaction to Taxol. She was a borderline diabetic and the glucose they gave her with the Taxol had triggered her diabetes. She had terrible side effects, so they switched her to Taxotere. She finished her series of chemo and six weeks of radiation and was put on Tamoxifen. Thankfully, Joyce is still cancer free today.

On March 24, 2000 I had my sixth and final round of chemotherapy. As a wonderful surprise I received an incredible bouquet of flowers from my son, Michael, to celebrate the end of the series of treatments. He has always been so thoughtful about the little things. During my radiation treatments when I first had cancer, he sent me a beautiful music box. Then, when those treatments were over I received a wonderful arrangement of flowers.

Receiving those flowers meant so much to me, that I try to remember to send flowers to friends I know who have completed their treatments or had surgery. When the cancer first metastasized in my liver, my gynecologist (whom I had only seen twice before) sent me a wonderful basket of flowers. That really blew me away and I still remember it with fondness. It brings real meaning to the phrase "the little things are what matter."

My stepson, David, was a junior in high school, and it was time for him to take a trip to look at the colleges he wanted to attend. He was interested in schools on the East Coast, so Michael and David planned a college trip back there during his spring break. I was disappointed that I couldn't go along, but it was right when my white count would be low, and travel would be out of the question for me. Cheryl came over from Tucson to stay with me while Michael went back East with David. They went to see Yale, Harvard, Penn, Princeton, Brown, Columbia, and Amherst.

Cheryl and I had fun, and even went out to lunch at the restaurant that would put us in a room by ourselves, so I didn't have to worry about germs. Mattie was also such a comfort and would snuggle next to me on the bed when I wasn't feeling quite up to par. I should probably have sent out a letter to all of Cheryl's patients thanking them for all the time she spent with me rather than with them! Len was also supportive of all the trips Cheryl made to be with me in Santa Barbara.

Michael and David returned home and brought back pictures of the schools they had visited. Yale was David's favorite, followed by Penn and Amherst. I was most impressed by Yale, although they were all quite amazing. We had always told David that if he could get accepted into the college of his choice, we would somehow find the money to pay for it, no matter where it was.

"You have to have confidence in your ability, and then be tough enough to follow through."

— ROSALYNN CARTER

CHAPTER FOUR

Hormone Therapy and the Avon 3-Day Walk

It was mid April, and I had finished my six cycles of chemotherapy. Now it was time to have another CT scan and see what effect the chemotherapy drugs had had on the tumors. The results would dictate what treatments were to follow. One thing I hoped for was that I would be able to try another type of chemo that didn't cause hair loss, so that I could finally let my hair grow. I was getting tired of wearing a wig.

The scan showed no change in the size of the tumors from the scan that had been done two months earlier. There were no new lesions, but the tumors in my liver didn't appear to have gotten any smaller. Even though the CT scan showed no improvement, a blood test showed that the liver enzymes were much improved. And, the level of activity of the cancer in my system as tracked by the tumor markers (CA15-3) was now at 128.6—down from 848 when the cancer first metastasized in my liver. Dr. Woliver said he would like me to go off chemotherapy entirely since it wasn't reducing the tumors, and start on hormone therapy instead. He explained there had been some great results with a hormone called Arimidex, which was an aromatase inhibitor. These drugs work to lower estrogen in the body and have been effective with tumors like mine that are estrogen sensitive. There would be relatively few side effects. I would not lose my hair, there would be no mouth sores, and my white blood cell count should not be effected. There was only a one percent chance that I would lose my eyebrows and eyelashes. I thought this sounded great, as it would give my body a chance to recover from the toxic drugs that had been pumped into my veins. The hormone would be taken in pill form. I liked that a great deal, because it would allow me to feel like my life was getting back to normal. I knew that I would still have to come in for an intravenous infusion of the bone-strengthening drug Aredia, but that would be for a much shorter length of time in the chemo room, and only once a month instead of every three weeks. I was scheduled to come back in 30 days for a blood test and an evaluation of how the Arimidex was working.

I realized much later—in December of 2004—how on top of the current research Dr. Woliver really was, when newspapers across the country started reporting about an amazing new cancer drug called Arimidex. It had been prescribed for me back in 2000!

Around this time, my son, Michael, came out to visit and wanted to meet Dr. Woliver. At that meeting (which was one week prior to our regularly scheduled appointment), I told Dr. Woliver that after three weeks of being on the hormone I had lost my eyebrows and eyelashes. I wasn't sure if this was a side effect from the final chemotherapy session, or was from the Arimidex. I had never lost my eyebrows and eyelashes during chemotherapy, but I wasn't sure if this was a delayed reaction. Dr. Woliver said he thought it was from the Arimidex. Unfortunately, I was in the one percent of patients who had that side effect. He switched me to another aromatase inhibitor, called Femara, that did not have loss of eyebrows and eyelashes as a side effect. Later I found a product called Underwear For Lashes® by Origins that really helped when my eyelashes grew back very thinly and not as dense. It finds every thin lash. It goes on white and then mascara goes on top and voila—I suddenly had lashes I didn't think were there!

Michael and I did a search on the internet for Femara and read some very encouraging reports. One of the great things about the internet is that there are some very good sites explaining various drugs. But, I still check with Dr. Woliver to be sure that the explanations are accurate.

During the appointment, my son asked to meet with Dr. Woliver alone and so I left the room. It was strange to have my son want to speak with my doctor without me being present. I think Dr. Woliver also felt a bit uncomfortable. But Michael later told me that he wanted to be blunt in asking the doctor about my prognosis, and he felt what the doctor might say could bother me. I think he was also afraid the doctor had not told me everything and therefore, he would have only heard what I had been told. This, of course, was not the case. Dr. Woliver had always been very up-front with me. I may have been a little gentle when I explained things to my son on the telephone, but the telephone is not the correct venue for such a sensitive subject. The good thing about his meeting with Dr. Woliver was that it opened up a dialogue between my son and me, so we could talk about everything in detail. We have always had a very close relationship and I was worried about how he would handle my cancer, but he has been extremely strong. He participates each year in the Relay for the Cure in Oregon. It is his way of being involved with trying to raise funds for cancer research. Soon after his visit, Michael passed the American Bar Association exam in Oregon and took a position as an assistant district attorney. I couldn't have been more proud, not just that he had passed the Bar exam, but that he had grown into a truly wonderful adult.

After my son went back to Oregon, all of the things we spoke about regarding my cancer and the possible outcomes played on my mind. I notice that I can be very strong, and actually rather detached, when I speak about my cancer. But at times when I am alone with my own thoughts, I get more emotional. Another trigger for my emotions is when I hear that someone has died of cancer. It doesn't matter if it is a celebrity or someone mentioned on the local news. I break down and cry for them, and I feel very vulnerable. These times do not linger, and I think it's healthy for me to get out emotions that I might otherwise stuff inside. It's detrimental to keep emotions all bottled up. I know that some people are afraid to get in touch with their feelings because they don't want to be out of control. For me, it's best to feel the fear and then let it go. Worrying or obsessing about the cancer and what the outcome will or will not be does not change the facts—it's quite simply non-productive.

Our next regular appointment with Dr. Woliver showed that Femara appeared to be keeping me stable. My tumor markers were even down from 128.6 to 79.6. This was the first time that my CA15-3 was below 100 (according to the lab I used, the normal range was 0-31.3). I was also feeling great. My hair was starting to grow in a tiny bit, and I was having no adverse side effects from the Femara. Food was starting to taste normal again, and what a pleasure it was not to have to worry about my white cell count. This was the best I had felt in a very long time.

Everything seemed great until I went in for my next infusion of Aredia and they couldn't find a vein to use for the I.V. That was very unsettling! I went into Dr. Woliver's office and asked him if Aredia or a similar drug came in tablet form. I was sick and tired of all of the needles. He said that actually it did come in a tablet by the name of Clodronate. Unfortunately, it was only available in Canada, Mexico and Europe. Dr. Woliver said that Clodronate (in Canada it's called Bonefos) had great promise and he expected it would soon be available in the U. S. Thus far there has been no comparative studies of Clodronate versus Zometa or Aredia, but they are all in the class of drugs referred to as bisphosphonates also called diphosphonates. Nonetheless, the data available from Europe suggests it's similar to infused Aredia and Zometa. I researched and located a pharmacy that carried Clodronate. I have found that cancer patients are only too willing to share information with other patients on where they get medicines, etc. I placed my order and was thrilled to be able to cancel my next I.V. infusion of Aredia. I knew that there was a possibility I would have to go back on I.V. chemo at a later date, and I wanted to save what veins I had left. It is important to point out that there is a risk when taking any of the bisphosphonates of getting a bone disease called Osteonecrosis of the Jaw (ONJ). This is something you should discuss with your oncologist.

It was May and time for the greeting card industry's biggest trade show—The National Stationary Show, which is held annually in New York City. I felt that I was too recently off chemotherapy to attend and so I sent two of my employees to work the show. I was on the Executive Committee of the Greeting Card Association's Board of Directors and since they needed a quorum for their meeting, they set up a conference call so I could sit in long distance. I had always considered it an honor to sit on such an important committee along with representatives from companies like Hallmark, American Greetings, Avanti, etc. It was nice to be from a small company and feel on an equal footing with the major players in the industry. Our cards also won several awards that year in the International Greeting Card Awards competition. I had always enjoyed attending that awards dinner and seeing the people I knew I was going to miss that.

I started my greeting card company, which was named EthnoGraphics, from my garage in 1987. The first cards showed just my photography, but the company eventually grew to publish the work of 75 artists and photographers from all over the world. We operated out of 6,500 square feet of warehouse and office space in an industrial area near the beach in Santa Barbara. We were the largest ethnic (multicultural) greeting card company in the industry. All of our artists were from the culture for which they created art—African American, Latino, Jewish, Asian and Native American. We also produced a line of animal cards and had a wonderful selection of multicultural cards depicting people from various cultures coming together. I felt very proud that our company filled an important niche in the marketplace.

In June, the Avon 3-Day Walk that Cheryl and I had signed up for started to loom on the horizon. I began getting all sorts of information in the mail about the proper way to train for the 60-mile event. The walk would take place in October and I knew I had to start doing some serious training. I had been walking regularly on my treadmill, but now I needed to do some outdoor training as well. I started taking daily walks with Mattie. My offices were only two blocks from the ocean, so we would go down to the beach and follow it up to the campus of Santa Barbara City College, and then back—a distance of about four miles. I then found that if we went past the street where my office was and continued to the Santa Barbara Zoo before turning back, we would get in six miles. That was a good distance for building up our endurance. Mattie was so cute as she trotted alongside me, her little legs going as fast as they could, but she easily kept up. My veterinarian was thrilled that Mattie was getting so much exercise, because Dachshunds have a tendency to get overweight. This was a great opportunity to just take in the beauty of Santa Barbara and have fun with Mattie.

Besides the training walks, I had to focus on raising the $1,500 in pledges that were required. Before my cancer metastasized, Michael and I would play golf. I stopped playing golf when I started wearing a wig because I was fearful that the wig would fly off when I swung the club. But I called the golf pro who had given us lessons (who also happened to be the general manager of the club) and explained that I was going to be doing the Avon 3-Day Walk. I asked if the club would perhaps sponsor me.

He suggested that instead they hold a golf tournament in my name and donate the proceeds. It was so nice of them. I soon raised the required $1,500, and eventually raised a total of $5,000.

Everything seemed to be going so well. My hair was growing back and was even curly. Some people call it "chemo" curl. I had heard it might not stay curly, but it was fun for the time being. It made losing my hair worth it! The good news carried through to my tumor markers, which went to a new low of 47.

That's when I developed an unexpected pain and numbness in my right hand. I was concerned this might be a side effect of Femara. When Dr. Woliver examined me, he explained that I had classic symptoms of carpal tunnel syndrome, and he referred me to a neurologist for further diagnosis. The neurologist conducted a series of very painful tests, sticking needles into my muscles and attaching them to a machine that confirmed that I did in fact have carpal tunnel syndrome in my right wrist.

I remember just sucking it up and allowing him to complete the tests, because he kept talking about how most men who came in for these tests were sissies and that they couldn't put up with what a woman like me could. He went on to tell me that he thought I would probably have to have surgery. First, however, he wanted me to try a new anti-inflammatory drug called Celebrex. He said it might relieve the rather intense pain and numbness I had been having. I thought it would be fine because I had never had problems with other anti-inflammatory medications, like advil or motrin.

Soon after starting the new medication, I developed a very bad pain in my abdomen. It was similar to the pain I had felt when the cancer first metastasized in my liver. We were afraid that suddenly the cancer had taken off again—with a vengeance! I made an immediate appointment with Dr. Woliver. When he asked if I had taken anything new, Michael spoke up and said I was taking a new anti-inflammatory drug. He told me to go off it and see what happened. The pain went away immediately. I have never been so relieved. I found out later that abdominal pain is a well documented side effect of Celebrex—something that I wish the neurologist who prescribed it would have mentioned. I also heard after this episode that those with liver disease should not take Celebrex! When those of us who have cancer experience an unexplained ache or pain, it is very common to immediately think that the cancer has spread, rather than looking towards a simple explanation, like an adverse reaction to a new medication.

The pain in my right hand and wrist was still very bad, and I wasn't sure what to do about it. I knew that I didn't want to go through surgery if it wasn't absolutely necessary. The surgery itself would be painful, and there would be an extended recovery period of up to six months. By coincidence, I opened the local paper and saw an ad from a chiropractor regarding treatments for carpal tunnel syndrome. It dawned on me that I had been treated for severe pain in my neck by a great chiropractor several years before. He worked with many athletes in Santa Barbara, using various methods that included acupressure and acupuncture. If any chiropractor could take care of carpal tunnel syndrome, then I felt that Dr. Thomas Rook could. At my first appointment, he confirmed that I did have carpal tunnel. Then, after a series of treatments, the pain went away completely and has never returned. Those painless treatments were better by far than having to go through surgery.

I was starting to feel like my hair was long enough so that I could go on my training walks with Mattie minus the wig. It was extremely short, but I was so tired of the wig. I decided that people could just stare if they wanted to. It wasn't until I saw a picture that was taken one month later in July at a family reunion in Missouri, that I realized how short it really was. But all of my husband's relatives at the reunion said it looked great.

They liked it, so I felt fine. I think because my hair is so blond that it looked even shorter, almost not there at all. I believe now that it was important for me to lose my hair, because I learned a lot about myself during that time. I have always felt that we need to learn lessons from the things that occur in life. When I got cancer I remember saying to myself, "Okay, what am I supposed to take away from this experience?"

Once when I was traveling, I showed my driver's license for ID, which had a photo from before the chemotherapy. Two security people looked at the photo and mentioned that my hair looked great long. I just thanked them and said that I had lost it in chemotherapy. They both were taken aback, and said that it looked great short too, and that more importantly I looked healthy. That really is the more important issue, isn't it?

In September, Cheryl, Len, Michael and I decided we needed to get away from all the medical stuff. We checked out several places and decided to go to the Banff Springs Hotel near Calgary in Canada, for a few days of rest and relaxation. The entire area was honestly one of the most spectacular places on earth. The views were breathtaking and the hotel was like a castle. We played golf, hiked, and took in all of the sights. Caribou were all over the place, including the golf course, where they were allowed to roam at will. We loved it! I was able to relax for the first time since the cancer treatments began. Cheryl and I also got in some training walks for the Avon 3-Day. It was very brisk out and so I bought some wonderful hats to cover my very cold head. At the end of our stay, we were all very sad to leave.

It was the beginning of October, 2000 and time for another CT scan and blood work-up. The tumor markers measured at 33.6—almost in the normal range of 31.3 or lower! The CT scan showed that the lesions in my liver were a bit smaller and there were fewer of them, so clearly I would be staying on Femara. I asked Dr. Woliver what the average time someone stayed on Femara, and he said around nine months. He also felt that the Clodronate I had been taking to strengthen my bones was having some positive influence on the cancer in my liver.

I couldn't have been happier with the results, and felt that I was in good shape to do the upcoming 3-day walk. I knew I would be doing 20 miles a day. Even though I had only gotten up to eight miles in my training walks, I felt fairly well prepared. After all, as they pointed out in the training bulletins, you only had to do 20 miles a day on the weekend of the walk itself.

Cheryl flew over from Tucson the morning before the walk and we spent the day getting registered, going through all of the required safety talks, and getting our tent. It was raining lightly, but that didn't put a damper on anything. It was so exciting seeing all of the women (and some men as well) who had come from all over to participate. There were over 3,000 walkers. It was very emotional seeing all the families that were walking together. There were mothers and daughters, sisters and brothers, aunts and uncles, as well as husbands, sons and fathers all walking for a loved one who either had cancer or had died from cancer.

Several months before the walk Cheryl and I had been interviewed over the telephone for an article they said would appear in the daily publication that would be handed out at the walk. The walking coach assigned to us had set it up, thinking it would be interesting to do an article about twins walking together. We had actually both forgotten about the whole thing, but there it was this first morning of the walk. Everyone was reading the article and asking if we were the twins it was written about. Cheryl and I enjoyed reading the article, and it opened up dialogue with many of the other walkers. Seeing me looking healthy and able to walk, while having fourth stage breast cancer was—I was told—inspiring to many of the other walkers. It was at this walk that I first realized it was important for me to speak openly about my cancer.

That first day of the walk, I met another cancer survivor named Angela Rooney. She was going through chemotherapy for metastasized cancer of the cervix (technically, adenocarcinoma of the cervix). She was so friendly and full of energy, and we hit it off immediately. She was walking with her brother and would not be staying in the "tent city" that was set up at night for all the walkers, since her immune system had been compromised by her chemotherapy. Her goal was simply to walk on all three days.

During the time we spent walking, she told me that she had heard about a medical doctor in Paris, France. A friend of her brother's was seeing him for cancer treatments. Angela, herself, was scheduled to see this doctor a couple of weeks after the walk. She told me that he was a medical doctor who prescribed plant-based medications, based on the results of a global diagnosis of the entire body. I found this very intriguing, and Angela said she would email me more information after the walk. Angela had first been diagnosed with cancer in 1999, at the age of 33. Although our cancers were different, our stories were similar in many ways. She was younger than me and had two small children, but the fact we were both fighting cancer created a bond between us. Neither of us had paper or pen to write down our email addresses, but fortunately she remembered mine and did email me after the walk to tell me all about her trip to Paris.

As Cheryl and I walked the last mile into camp the first day of the walk, we were so surprised to see Len waiting for us. He not only walked the last mile with us; he helped set up our tent. He and Michael had decided they would each come during different stages to root us on. Actually, I was blown away by all the people lining the route each day of the walk. They had signs, candy, and many were dressed in creative costumes to encourage every walker to make that next mile.

During the first day, a pebble in my shoe had created a blister on the heel of my right foot, so after getting into camp, I showered and went over to the medical tents that were set up to deal with blisters, pulled muscles, sprained ankles, etc. There were so many emergency room doctors, chiropractors, physical therapists, and massage therapists who volunteered their time to help the walkers each day. Since we had gotten into camp early that day, I was quickly attended to by the medical personnel. Later the lines were very long. My foot got all taped up and I was ready for the second day of the walk. I also saw one of the physical therapists who worked on my sore muscles to keep them loose. Cheryl and I both felt great after the first day.

At the camp there was a huge circus-like tent where food was served cafeteria style. Everyone ate at long tables inside the tent. There was an amazing number of volunteers who did the cooking and serving, and set up all of the tables. After the meal, we rested in our tent and went back later to check out the entertainment that was going on. It was fun, but the best thing was spending time with Cheryl, just talking in our tent. It was like camping out. We used a flashlight to get to the portable toilets in the middle of the night. We hadn't done that since we were small. She and I were the youngest of five children. Our parents took the family camping for every holiday break and summer vacations. During a couple of summers when we were in junior high and high school, we spent the entire summer in a tent while our father worked as a carpenter in a nearby town.

The second day of the walk Michael and David came to the park where we stopped for lunch. It was so much fun to see them, and we were feeling in great shape. They couldn't believe how wonderful we looked after walking 20 miles the day before and spending a night in a sleeping bag on the ground. It was a beautiful, sunny day. Michael mentioned that we were once again in the top part of the walk. He and David had been stationed at the park since the first walkers came through and we weren't far behind them.

We had so much fun walking that second day. I finished the day without too much trouble, but the blister on my heel was bothering me as we came into camp. So I showered and went over to get it checked out. The podiatrist who saw me said that the blister had spread over my entire heel and was much too severe for me to walk the next day (which was the final day of the walk). I let him know that I would be very upset if I couldn't finish the walk. He told me to come back in the morning at 6 am and he would check it again.

I went back to the tent and Cheryl held me while I cried. It meant so much for me to finish this walk. I was heartbroken at the thought of not being able to walk across the finish line holding Cheryl's hand. Both of us went to bed hoping the blister would miraculously be fine in the morning. I was the first person waiting at the medical tent at 6 am. Lucky for me, I ended up seeing an emergency room doctor from UCLA. I explained to her how important this walk was to me. I told her I didn't go through chemotherapy and all of the training not to finish. She was so sympathetic and she told me that she understood. She bandaged me up so that I was able to finish the walk. She knew this was an emotional thing and that it went far beyond medicine.

Off Cheryl and I went, but on this third day of the walk the rain started coming down hard and it stayed that way all day long. What a mess! Most people were not prepared for rain at all. It was a very unusual storm for Southern California at that time of year. Many walkers actually ended up wearing garbage bags as rain gear. Our shoes soon became soaked, as we had to walk through puddles throughout the day. Blisters became a big problem for practically everyone, because it was impossible to keep your feet dry. I went to one of the medical stations set up along the route to have a blister on my little toe taped and to have my heel checked.

At lunch Cheryl asked if I wanted to take the bus into the finish line. She was worried about my heel. I told her I wanted to try it a little longer.

There were vans going up and down the highway, asking all the walkers if they wanted a ride to the next stop or the finish line, but we said no thanks. We found ourselves walking with a group of women who were singing all sorts of songs—mostly oldies and songs from different musicals. That really perked us up. We joined in, and when they stopped, we started singing our college fight songs and songs we sang as children at Camp Fire Girls' camp. I don't know how in the world we ever remembered the words! We just kept going, mile after mile.

Then, as we were walking up Pacific Coast Highway, with the rain pouring down and the wind in our faces, we saw the finish line up ahead. That's when we knew we would be able to complete the walk on our own. What a sight! There had been so many people lining the highway cheering us on throughout the day, but now the crowd was enormous and it gave us all the push we needed to walk those last few miles.

Finally, we crossed the line and shook so many hands. We started looking for Michael and Len, but there were too many people everywhere and we couldn't see them. We had all arranged to meet at the closing ceremony, but both Cheryl and I were completely soaked and I was starting to shiver from the cold. I just wanted to get into a nice warm car. We didn't care if we went through the closing ceremony, but we had no choice, since that was where we knew we could find them. We had all tried using our cell phones, but so did 6,000 other people and so no phones would work. By this time I was shaking badly—probably from dehydration. All that day when we had been walking in the rain, we didn't want to stop and use a porta potty because we felt it would be too uncomfortable to pull down all that wet clothing. Therefore, we didn't drink nearly as much water as we should have.

Before the closing ceremony, all the walkers were given a new dry long-sleeve T-shirt to put on. But there were only a few places to stand out of the rain so they didn't stay dry for very long. I was given a pink shirt because I am a cancer survivor. Cheryl was given a blue one. All the women with pink shirts were asked to walk together in the middle of the group, but I refused because I wanted to walk with Cheryl. It was so bizarre. Everyone was trying to get all the walkers organized for a final walk through soaked sand and huge puddles of water into the area where the closing ceremony would take place. We were all so exhausted, and yet very excited that we had completed the 60 miles.

But, we were never so happy as the moment we finally saw our husbands near the end of the closing ceremony. We motioned for them to meet us around the side of the bleachers, and we got our luggage and rushed to the car. I have never been so thankful for heated seats! I pulled off all of my wet clothes and put on a warm, dry sweatshirt and pants. I turned the heat up high, and then realized I badly needed to rehydrate, so I started drinking as much water as I could. The shakes finally stopped as we drove into Santa Barbara. That last day was an ordeal, but there were also so many fond memories of the wonderful people Cheryl and I had met during the walk. We also felt we had accomplished what we had set out to do. That walk netted 6.6 million dollars for breast cancer research.

When I think back about that final day of the walk, I realize that it probably would have been smarter for me to have taken the bus to the finish line, as Cheryl had suggested at lunch. But, I guess that emotionally I just needed to finish the walk. As a result of the walk, I ended up losing many of my toenails, and I couldn't wear my shoes for weeks because of the blisters. I think 60 miles is a very long distance and I'm glad that Avon has now shortened it to a two-day walk. It's more manageable for most people—especially those who are actively fighting cancer and may be on chemotherapy. Nevertheless, right after the walk, Cheryl and I signed up for the next year hoping for sun.

Several weeks later, in December, my new friend Angela emailed me about her trip to Paris. She told me how impressed she was with the doctor she had seen there, Dr. Jean-Claude Lapraz. I told Michael that I thought it was too much of a coincidence that I had met Angela just before she went to Paris, and that my daughter, Kim, was living in Paris. I felt that I should also consider going to see Dr. Lapraz. Michael agreed completely. I emailed Angela and asked if she could give me an email address for Dr. Lapraz—that I was considering going to Paris to see him. She told me that she thought that he wasn't taking any new patients, but that his associate would probably be able to see me. (By the way, Angela has continued to see Dr. Lapraz and, to date, hasn't had a reoccurrence of her cancer. She remains in full remission).

I sent an email to Dr. Lapraz in late January making initial inquiries. He emailed me right back saying that, fortunately, he could see me and that I should come as soon as possible. He suggested we schedule an appointment for the week of February 10, 2001. Dr. Lapraz's email indicated that he was working in close cooperation with another physician, Dr. Christian Duraffourd, who had created a new approach to medicine that takes a patient's entire body into account. He suggested that perhaps this approach could help my body fight the disease. He continued,

> "With my colleague Dr. Duraffourd, we have been working for a long time in a Paris hospital dedicated to treating breast cancer in women, and our aim has been to help them to improve the efficiency and tolerance of their classical products, by using what has been named oncobiology. We have treated many people and many of them have obtained a better and longer life. I can receive you in France as soon as you can come."

He went on to ask for my medical records and he sent a list of what items he wanted included in a blood test. He ended his email with "Keep hope, we will try to help you in the best way we know." He signed it, "Best regards, Docteur J.C. Lapraz."

It was time to see Dr. Woliver and go over the results of my recent lab work. The news was not good. My tumor markers were going up—they had risen to 48.2. Dr. Woliver ordered a new CT scan so he could see what was going on. It showed a new, rather large tumor in my liver. It was clear that I had a progressive disease, and it was decided that I should stop taking Femara. I had been on Femara for ten months, which was about the average time I had been told that the hormone was usually effective for cancer patients with metastasized tumors. Dr. Woliver suggested I try another hormone, since hormone therapy had seemed to be effective for me. He prescribed one called Megace (progesterone).

At this appointment I explained to Dr. Woliver I was going to be traveling to see Dr. Lapraz in Paris, and that I would need copies of all of my medical records to forward to him. I explained that Dr. Lapraz treats the underlying dysfunctions of the body that generate disease in the first place, and that he uses plant-based medications to help patients improve their tolerance of conventional medicines. I felt that because Dr. Lapraz was a medical doctor, Dr. Woliver would feel more comfortable about my seeing him. As I have mentioned, Dr. Wolver seemed open to complementary treatments as long as he didn't feel they would compromise my health. Dr. Woliver suggested I wear support stockings on the flight, and get up and walk up and down the aisle frequently. Apparently blood clots were a common side effect of the medication I was taking.

After I picked up the copy of my medical records from Dr. Woliver's office, I decided to read all 80 pages before sending them off to Dr. Lapraz. Actually seeing the words "fourth stage breast cancer" really hit me hard. It's not that I didn't already know it—it's just that seeing it in print regarding my own diagnosis for the first time was difficult. As I sent the material off to Dr. Lapraz, I finally felt that I was taking control of my own body and doing what I needed to do in order to fight the cancer and improve the quality of my life.

"A strong positive mental attitude will create more miracles than any wonder drug."

—PATRICIA NEAL

CHAPTER FIVE

Meeting Dr. Jean-Claude Lapraz

Michael and I left for Paris on Sunday, February 11, 2001. Cheryl came as well, but Len was not able get away from his office. We were all very excited to be traveling to Paris, not only to see Dr. Lapraz, but also because we had not seen Kim in almost a year. We had originally planned to go to Paris and see Dr. Lapraz before I had the CT scan showing a new tumor in my liver. So, we felt that the timing was especially important.

After arriving at our hotel in Paris, we called Kim and she came right over. She looked great, and very French with her short bangs and Sasson style haircut. Since Kim was the only one of us who spoke French, we asked her to call Dr. Lapraz's office and let him know that we had arrived. Following his request, Kim then called the Paris lab where he wanted me to go for another blood draw and made an appointment for nine the next morning. I knew that, for some reason, the lab in Santa Barbara had not been able to do all of the tests that Dr. Lapraz wanted—even though Dr. Woliver had explained each of them to the lab technician.

We looked at a map of the wonderful Paris subway system (the Metro) and saw that there were stops close to both the lab and to Dr. Lapraz's office. We would be seeing Dr. Lapraz in the afternoon, shortly after the lab appointment. Kim was a huge help on this trip, for she knew Paris fairly well. She taught us the ins and outs of the Metro system, and how the city is divided into districts. I had only been to Paris for a few days many years before.

Our art deco style hotel was charming. It was located on Boulevard Haussmann in the Opera District, and was only a 15-minute walk from the Louvre. We discovered that many wonderful restaurants and cafés were also just a few short blocks away. Paris most definitely does not lack in places to go for great food. We found that walking is the best way to really "see" the city. At the hotel, Michael and I had a room that adjoined Cheryl's room, so it felt like our family had a little suite. From our balcony you could see the Eiffel Tower off in the distance. While it was nice to get out and do some sightseeing, I was very anxious about my meeting with Dr. Lapraz. I could hardly sleep that night.

In the morning we went right over to the lab. Kim served as our translator because no one there spoke English. The woman who took my blood asked Kim if her job was to take Americans around to doctors appointments and act as their translator. Kim was very amused by that! After leaving the lab, we were all very hungry. We found a great little café, called the Coppernic, a few blocks away and within sight of the Arc de Triomphe. They really knew how to make wonderful fried eggs, and their bread was just amazing. Since that first trip, we have made it part of our regular routine to stop at the Coppernic café after going to the lab.

When we left the café we walked over to the Arc de Triomphe and then down the Avenue des Champs Elysées. There is nothing quite like walking down the Champs Elysées. It's a wide boulevard full of great shops to cruise through. There are cafés and restaurants galore filled with wonderful places to sit, have a cappuccino or glass of wine, and watch the amazing parade of people strolling by.

That day, we were all a bundle of nerves and full of excitement before our initial meeting with Dr. Lapraz. Angela had sent me a picture of her with Dr. Lapraz, so I did know what he looked like. But I later found that his very genuine warmth could only be felt in person. Kim came with us to the appointment in case we needed a translator, but that turned out to be unnecessary since Dr. Lapraz's English was quite good.

So, at the appointed time Cheryl, Michael, Kim, and I took the Metro to Dr. Lapraz's office. It was located on a tree-lined street in a nice district of Paris. We made ourselves comfortable in the reception room and waited for what seemed liked an eternity. Then, he suddenly popped in and introduced himself. His bright smile and relaxing manner immediately put me at ease. He invited all four of us to come back to his office, and a whole new phase of my life began.

During that first meeting, Dr. Lapraz asked a lot of questions about the state of my health in general, and about my childhood. One of his questions was why the surgeon who removed the tumor from my breast had only taken eight lymph nodes for analysis to see if the cancer had spread. He pointed out that in France, they would have removed at least 25. He felt that eight lymph nodes were too few to test in order to determine that the cancer had not spread into my lymph system. This was the first time I had heard that an insufficient number of lymph nodes had been taken, and I made a mental note to check it out when we got back to Santa Barbara. He also questioned why my tumor markers had not been followed by my original oncologist, since only eight lymph nodes had been taken. He saw that it would have been easy to follow the tumor markers since I was going in for blood work every three to four months. I had already been wondering about that myself, and decided to ask Dr. Woliver about it when we got back. We spoke for more than two hours. I was so impressed with his engaging manner—you most definitely felt he listened with great interest to every word spoken, and he wrote everything down.

After our conversation, Dr. Lapraz gave me a very thorough physical examination. He felt so deeply into the tissue that, at times it was rather painful. But I felt confident that it was necessary, because of the way he explained what he was doing and what he was looking for. He told me that in probing various parts of the body, he was searching for the ending nerve points of organs in order to assess their state of inflammation. He was also examining things such as the condition of the skin, the nails, the hair, the iris of the eyes, reflex points, etc. It was the sort of examination that few doctors seem to perform today.

Dr. Lapraz made a point of saying that he wanted to work as part of a team with my Santa Barbara oncologist in treating me. I liked that a great deal. I think if he had made me feel like I had to choose between his treatments and what I was doing in Santa Barbara, I would have been very concerned. He also told me that he would create a report on his findings for Dr. Woliver, including what medicines he wanted me to take and why. Dr. Lapraz also mentioned that he had been working with other patients whose cancer had spread to their liver, and that many of them had been living for quite a number of years. This was a very different scenario than the one I had heard in the States.

I learned that Dr. Lapraz and his colleague, Dr. Christian Duraffourd, were both medical doctors who had been in general practice for more than 30 years. For eight of those years they worked solely as oncobiologists at a hospital in Paris, specializing in the treatment of cancer. A few years before my first appointment with Dr. Lapraz, he and Dr. Duraffourd had gone into private practice in order to work with patients on a preventive basis, as well as continuing to work with patients whose disease had progressed. In the hospital, they had mainly worked with patients whose cancers were already in advanced stages. This had allowed them to realize the secondary effects of chemotherapy and radiation. But, they wanted to do more, and hoped to help patients before their disease became advanced.

Both doctors had been disappointed by the limited ability of conventional medical science to deal with pathologies like cancer. They felt that traditional medicine was based on too standardized an approach, utilizing very rigid protocols that did not take the patient's background into account. Over the past 20 years, Doctors Lapraz and Duraffourd conceived and designed a different approach to medicine, which they refer to as endobiogénie. It's a global approach to the health of the patient, as opposed to the traditional approach, which is purely symptomatic. Endobiogénie looks at the body as a single system managed by the neuro-endocrine system. That is the system of glands, such as the thyroid, thymus and pituitary that, when stimulated by the nervous system, secrete hormones that regulate or influence other organs in the body.

Also at that first meeting, Dr. Lapraz told Cheryl that, since she was my identical twin, he would like her to get a blood test so he could see how she was doing. Recent research has shown that women who have an identical twin sister with breast cancer are four times more likely than average to develop it themselves. He said if there was something in the results he was concerned about, he could treat her preventively. So the next day we would go back to the lab for Cheryl's blood to be drawn. We all left his office with a great feeling, he was such a gentle soul with a very positive attitude—as well as being extremely knowledgeable. I felt he was someone I could trust completely, and that he would play a very important role in my battle with breast cancer. We ended that first lengthy session by making an appointment for the following Friday evening at 8 pm. At that appointment he would go over the results of the lab work with us, and prepare a prescription for the medicines I would need to take. I was truly impressed and could tell that he was an extremely dedicated doctor. He made it very clear that I should schedule another trip to Paris to see him in three months so he could monitor my progress closely. After that, he said he thought that we would be able to spread the appointments out to every six months.

We had three days before our next appointment with Dr. Lapraz, so we played tourist with Kim as our guide. We went to every museum we could fit in. Michael wanted to go to the Louvre and Kim didn't, so she met us later at the Musée d'Orsay, a beautifully renovated railway station that was built in 1900. The museum is filled with wonderful works by Monet, Renoir, Degas, Manet, and other artists of the late 19th and early 20th centuries. We ate lunch at an elegant restaurant there, sitting in front of huge windows that looked out over the rooftops of Paris. We also visited the Pompidou Center, France's national museum of modern art. The building itself is like a work of art, and it houses another unique restaurant.

It was nice to get away from the medical stuff for a few days and just relax and take in all the incredible sights of one of the most beautiful cities in the world. It worked out that we were there for Valentine's Day, and there couldn't be a more romantic city to be celebrating it in. I felt badly that Cheryl was there without Len, but he sent her a gorgeous bouquet of red roses that arrived at our hotel on Valentine's Day. That really cheered her up. We also spent an evening visiting Kim in her loft apartment in the Montparnasse area on the Left Bank. It was such great fun going with her to one of her favorite restaurants.

Before we knew it, it was Friday night and time for our second appointment with Dr. Lapraz. After we all went over the results of the blood work, he asked his colleague, Dr. Duraffourd, to join us. Dr. Lapraz wanted Dr. Duraffourd to examine me, and I agreed. They conversed in French during the exam, as Dr. Duraffourd doesn't speak English. It appeared to me that they were in complete agreement about my diagnosis. Dr. Lapraz then translated what he and Dr. Duraffourd had been saying, and confirmed that this was the case.

Dr. Lapraz explained that they had determined I had an overabundance of estrogen and progesterone in my body and that, when I was prescribed hormone replacement drugs containing estrogen and progestin, my body didn't know what to do with the excess hormones. Those excess hormones were the catalyst for the formation of the tumor or, at the very least, fed the tumor that was already there. This was precisely what I had suspected. I realized then that my gynecologist should have ordered a blood test before she prescribed the hormone replacement tablets. I remember that I didn't have hot flashes, which I had told her at the time. Now I knew why I hadn't had hot flashes—my body was saturated with estrogen! But, in 1996, what my doctor did was accepted practice by most gynecologists. My hope is that common practice today would be to order a blood test first, before hormone therapy is even considered. I had only been on the hormones for about a year when the tumor appeared.

Dr. Lapraz told me the blood work showed that my tumor markers (CA15-3) were up to 69.5—considerably higher than they had been the week before, when blood tests were performed in Santa Barbara. (The normal range for the CA15-3 at the Paris lab was 0-28.) Because there was an overabundance of progesterone in my system, he wanted me to go off Megace (the hormone therapy I had been taking) immediately. It was only adding more progesterone to my body. I had actually been concerned about taking Megace, so I had no problem with stopping it. Dr. Lapraz also explained that my thyroid was not working properly. I told him that it had seemed impossible for me to lose weight. He said that I could have been starving myself and still would not have lost weight, because my thyroid was virtually shut down. I was finally starting to get some answers.

We saw that Dr. Lapraz entered all of my blood results into a computer program. He explained that this diagnostic tool had originally been designed by Dr. Duraffourd, and was based on the work they had done together at Hospital Boucicault ten years before. It lets a doctor visualize a patient's biological functions through a spreadsheet displaying over 150 indices. These indices quantify the state of the functions that control the entire system (endocrine glands, circulating hormones, organs, etc.). Dr. Lapraz selected a few of these indices and explained to us what they meant. He referred to this diagnostic tool as the "Biology of Functions."

I had never been exposed to this kind of an overall view of the way the body works as a unified organism. Since it contains quantified information on so many different aspects of the body's inner workings, the Biology of Functions can monitor the state of a person's health over time. It was easy for me to understand how this could be an important tool in preventative medicine. As we discussed preventative medicine, Dr. Lapraz used illnesses that are caused by germs as an example. He explained that our bodies naturally contain many germs, but by treating the general state of our bodies we can prevent the activation and proliferation of those germs. He referred to the state of an individual's body as that person's terrain. In this view, treating the patient's terrain and bringing their body into balance is what preventative medicine is all about. This same approach also applies to degenerative diseases like cancer, which are often the result of internal dysfunctions. By controlling the state of the terrain of our bodies, we can reduce the risk that pathologies such as cancer would ever appear in the first place.

To better understand how each person's individual terrain affects their health, imagine that ten people—all dressed the same way—are exposed to extreme cold. Those ten people will all react differently. One may get sinusitis, two others pneumonia, a fourth might come down with rheumatic fever, and the fifth could get an acute eye inflammation. The remaining five might get nothing at all. The difference is that the terrain of each individual reacts to the cold in a different way.

The terrains of our bodies are rarely perfect. Sometimes we meet people who are under heavy stress, yet appear to be in good shape. These people probably belong to the 15 percent of the population who have a naturally balanced terrain. They have to expend little energy in order to maintain that balance. Of course, they will eventually die like everybody else, but they will die in relatively good shape. The remaining 85 percent of us have to fight to maintain a balanced terrain, exerting great energy in the process. As long as we have energy to spare, we will manage. But when our energy gets low, disease will appear.

One of the forerunners of modern medicine was a French biologist named Louis Pasteur who discovered that infections are caused by germs. This created a whole new world of opportunities to treat pathologies. If you could kill the germ, you would get rid of the sickness. The benefits were extraordinary. It seemed that people would no longer die from infections. With the goal of killing germs, modern chemistry was able to extract active ingredients from plants and make medications that were up to a thousand times stronger than the natural substances.

But this oversimplification (sickness = symptoms = germs) has its limits. There are millions of germs in our bodies at any given time, and most of them are inactive. If, for example, a germ proliferates because the pancreas is not functioning properly, you could kill the germ with antibiotics and get rid of the sickness. But, the patient is still left with a malfunctioning pancreas. The germ, like a Phoenix, will rise from its ashes and reappear a few months later. The malfunctioning pancreas is the issue, not the germ. The terrain of the body must be balanced to allow the pancreas to function correctly.

I had heard of homeopathy and asked Dr. Lapraz if his methods were similar. He explained that the homeopathic approach is actually quite different. Homeopathy is aimed at triggering reactions in the body by recreating—at very low levels—the symptoms of the disease being treated. It is, therefore, a symptomatic approach. Unlike Drs. Duraffourd and Lapraz's methods, it moves directly from symptoms to treatment, without addressing the physiological root causes of the symptoms.

We spoke with Dr. Lapraz in his office for several hours. After answering all of our questions, he wrote a prescription for the medicines he wanted me to start taking. Their goal was to get my body back into balance. He also told me he wanted me to eliminate all dairy, soy, and wheat from my diet. Dairy was to be eliminated because proteins in dairy products tend to stimulate inflammation and generate allergies through the production of immunoglobulins. They also produce cholesterol which is transformed into estrogen. Wheat can have an effect similar to dairy products by stimulating the production of immunoglobulins and creating allergies. I was to eliminate soy from my diet because it contains estrogen. Eating foods high in estrogen was definitely not a good idea, since I had a disease aggravated by an excess of it.

I had been a vegetarian for many years, and had only recently started eating fish in order to get more protein. I now decided to also add poultry to my diet, since I was going to be eliminating soy. Dr. Lapraz mentioned that red wine would be good in moderation (a glass at dinner), but not white. So red wine also became a part of my new diet.

A substance known as trans-Resveratrol (often called Res) which has cancer-fighting properties, is found in red grapes. Some people use the phrase "French paradox" when referring to the fact that the French have lower rates of heart disease and some cancers, despite a national diet high in fat. Compared to others in Europe, the French eat more beef, cheese, butter and other artery-clogging foods, but they also drink more red wine. Researchers have speculated that certain compounds in grapes, and grape products like red wine, offer some kind of protection from the negative effects of a high-fat diet. I have also heard that certain substances unique to wine, such as tannins and flavonoids, act as antioxidants. They may be key factors in the positive effects of red wine consumption. It all sounded good to me! If I were going to be giving up dairy products, I would at least be able to enjoy a glass of red wine.

Most of the medicines (which were all made from plants) that Dr. Lapraz prescribed were liquids that would come to me in small bottles. I was to use a dropper supplied by the Paris pharmacy that prepared the medicines in order to measure out the proper dosage from each bottle. I would then put the prescribed amount of each of six liquids into a glass of warm water and drink the combination before each meal. I was also told to drink one liter of tea made from a special mixture of dried herbs every day. The pharmacy would also supply those dried herbs.

As he was explaining all the medicines I would have to take, Dr. Lapraz casually mentioned that I would also have to give myself injections on a regular basis. They would be injections of an extract from the mistletoe plant, and he told me they would build up my immune system. I was to give myself an injection every other day for two weeks, and then lay off for two weeks. As he spoke, the color drained from my face. I told him I didn't think I could do it. I was upset at the thought of having to give myself a shot, but he calmly took out a syringe and showed me how to give myself an injection in my thigh. I was amazed because it didn't hurt at all. It was only a subcutaneous injection, like many diabetics give themselves every day. It was clear then and there, that I was going to have to get over my fear of needles.

Dr. Lapraz said he would fax the prescription to the pharmacy and that they would have a three-month supply of the medicines ready for us to pick up the next evening. There are phytotherapic and homeopathic pharmacies all over Paris—very different from what one would find in the United States.

After explaining everything to me, Dr. Lapraz told Cheryl that the results of her blood tests had not come back yet, and that he would call her in Tucson to go over them. Then he said his goodbyes and told me to have courage. He has ended many of his emails to me with "Continuez a combattre avec courage" (Continue to fight with courage). Dr. Lapraz is full of concern for each and every one of his patients. I feel lucky to be one of them.

The next night Michael went alone to pick up the medicines at the pharmacy because I wasn't feeling well. Poor Michael—he came back to the hotel loaded down with two huge bags filled with bottles, vials and a large box of loose tea. Now, we had to find a way to fit them all into our suitcases!

While we were still in Paris, I started to get very angry about the fact that my tumor markers had not been followed by my first oncologist. I also thought about the fact that the surgeon who removed my tumor had only taken eight lymph nodes for testing. My cancer had gone from stage one to stage four in less than two years, while none of the well-respected medical professionals I had been seeing regularly noticed its progression. I felt that I should have known more back then, so that I could have questioned the actions of the surgeon and oncologist right from the beginning. I finally let go of the anger. Anger wasn't going to change anything—it was just a waste of energy. I'm sure that most of us play the "what if" game. What if I hadn't gone on hormone replacement drugs? What if they had taken more lymph nodes and found that the cancer had spread, and then treated it more aggressively? What if my first oncologist had followed the tumor markers, noticed they were going up, and started the chemotherapy sooner?

But the "what if" game doesn't change the facts. What was happening right then was what I had to deal with. My energies had to be used to fight the cancer. Then I would be able to figure out how to let other people know what type of questions they should ask their doctors, so that my experiences would not have been in vain. While I was frustrated by the past, I was rejuvenated and extremely excited about starting a new phase of my life. I would be working to get my body back into balance with the help of Drs. Lapraz and Duraffourd and the plant-based medicines.

"Nothing in life is to be feared. It is only to be understood."

—MARIE CURIE

CHAPTER SIX

Xeloda and My Second Trip to Paris

We returned home from Paris with a suitcase full of medicines that filled our pantry. Michael was a great help in organizing all of the bottles. I found that it took anywhere from 15 minutes to a half hour three times a day just to measure out and drink the concoction (which did not taste good at all), count out the tablets, make the tea and do the injection. Actually, Michael usually gets up and brews the tea for me because it's supposed to brew for 20 minutes, and he's up early. But this was my life we were trying to save, and we were both willing to do whatever it took.

Two weeks after returning from Paris, I had an appointment with Dr. Woliver. At this appointment I explained that Drs. Duraffourd and Lapraz wanted me to go off the Megace he had prescribed, because they had discovered my body had an overabundance of progesterone. Although they told me to stop taking Megace (a hormone therapy), the doctors in Paris had encouraged me to go on chemotherapy to kill the cancer cells in my body.

Dr. Woliver was fine with the fact that I had stopped taking Megace. He said the pills were obviously not doing anything for me since my tumor markers had gone up after starting them. In fact, the new blood test I took in Santa Barbara after returning from Paris showed the tumor markers had climbed even higher.

I was anxious to know what Dr. Woliver's next step would be. We spoke about Dr. Lapraz's treatment plan and I gave Dr. Woliver a copy of the prescription he had written. Dr. Woliver seemed very interested. I told him that Dr. Lapraz was preparing a report that would explain the treatments I had been put on. I also mentioned that Dr. Lapraz wanted to work with him as part of a team.

We then spoke about what type of chemo I would go on next. Dr. Woliver told me about a new chemotherapy drug called Xeloda. It was taken in tablet form. He told me it had been used with great success for patients whose cancer had metastasized in the liver. He went on to explain that the potential side effects were diarrhea, soreness, and blisters in the palms of the hands and on the bottom of the feet. But usually there were no problems with low white blood cell counts or loss of hair. Inside my head I was hollering "Yeah, no Neupogen shots and no hair loss!"

Dr. Woliver said he would start me on a lower dosage of Xeloda than the one recommended by the manufacturer. He explained that the toxicity of the full dose is often greater than many people can tolerate, and smaller doses are often as effective. I loved the idea of not having to go in for I.V. infusions, and that the side effects sounded manageable. I was to take three Xeloda tablets in the morning and two in the evening (each tablet is 500 mg), for a period of two weeks. Then I would be completely off the tablets for one week. I knew it was still chemotherapy, but taking it in tablet form made me feel as though I could go on living my life and this would just be part of the daily routine. It was a huge mental boost.

From the beginning, I was thrilled because I had very few side effects from Xeloda. I did notice that I would have to eat something more than just a piece of fruit in the morning when I took the tablets, or I would get a little queasy. The challenge for me was to find something I liked to eat since Dr. Lapraz had taken me off dairy, soy and wheat. I settled on peanut butter on bananas, or peanut butter on rice cakes. But that got old fast! We finally found a non-wheat bread made from a grain called spelt. I couldn't wait to taste it and made some toast as soon as we got home from the store. "Heavenly" is the word that comes to mind to describe that first bite! Dr. Lapraz had said that I could have four eggs a week, so an egg on a piece of my new spelt toast made a wonderful breakfast!

The only other side effect I had was after being on Xeloda for two weeks was diarrhea, but it was manageable. I don't know if the plant-based medicines prescribed by Dr. Lapraz reduced the side effects of Xeloda, or if I was just lucky. I know several other patients have had more severe side effects from the drug. I emailed Dr. Lapraz to tell him about the new drug that Dr. Woliver had prescribed. He wrote back to tell me that he was familiar with Xeloda and thought it would work well in conjunction with the plant-based medicines. Dr. Lapraz explained that the purpose of the medications he had prescribed was to improve the terrain of my body and increase my tolerance to chemo and other therapies.

As I have mentioned, Dr. Lapraz wanted me to eliminate dairy products from my diet. His explanation had sounded quite logical to me. Later I discovered the writings of Dr. Jane Plant, a professor and prominent scientist in England. Dr. Plant contracted breast cancer in 1987. She had five recurrences, and by 1993 the cancer had metastasized and she was given three months to live. She felt that it was time to take matters into her own hands and researched the damaging effects of dairy products in relation to breast cancer. She wrote a book called *Your Life in Your Hands: Understanding, Preventing and Overcoming Breast Cancer*. Many cancer patients have read and swear by it. It's a compelling story and I think she makes some interesting points regarding dairy.

In her book, Dr. Plant suggests substituting soy for dairy. But, I think a person should know if they have an overabundance of estrogen in their body before considering this. Soy naturally contains estrogen, which in large quantities may be harmful. In my case, it was important to eliminate soy from my diet. We all have completely different chemical make ups. Soy may be fine for some but not for others. That is why it's important to know the estrogen level in your body.

Giving up dairy products was the single hardest thing for me to do. I am a lover of cheese—any kind of cheese! If cheese was part of the description of an item on a restaurant menu, it always got my full attention. While I was a vegetarian, I was never a vegan. I found giving up meat very easy, but in earlier times giving up cheese would have been impossible for me. Today, I occasionally cheat and add some cheese to a salad, but rarely. Dr. Lapraz knew how difficult this was for me, and he said that one-day a month I could have as much cheese as I wanted. So, I decided that maybe a little bit of cheese every now and then would be about the same. Still, I know it's silly to think that I can't live without cheese. After all, I got cancer while not eating meat or drinking alcohol—two things I have heard that put a woman at increased risk of breast cancer. But when cheese was an important part of my diet, I did get breast cancer. Maybe there is something for me to think about here. I know that scientists associated with the National Dairy Council feel that Professor Plant's book is full of inaccuracies, but they obviously may have a conflict of interest regarding the consumption of dairy products. I don't profess to be an expert in this area, but I do believe it's worth finding out more about the dangers of dairy in relation to breast cancer. What's the downside of knowing the facts?

In March 2001 it was reported in the media that actress Suzanne Somers was taking homeopathic medicine to treat her breast cancer. She disclosed that a malignant tumor had been removed from her breast, and that she was injecting herself daily with a drug called Iscador—which is derived from the mistletoe plant. She said she planned to do this for five years and didn't want to go on chemotherapy. Since cancer hadn't been found in her lymph nodes, it made no sense to me that some people were quite distressed about the treatment she had chosen. I felt she was doing more, not less. She said that if her cancer spread, she would reconsider her decision about chemotherapy. I feel it's important for someone to make their own decision after carefully considering all the options. I applaud her for taking control of her own body. I'm sure that time will tell if this was a prudent decision or not.

Right after I heard about Suzanne Somers' mistletoe (Iscador) injections, I went to the Internet to research the substance that Dr. Lapraz had prescribed for me to inject myself with. I found that it was exactly the same thing. I had been injecting the mistletoe extract into my thigh. Sometimes I hit a muscle, which was quite painful. The research I read suggested that these sorts of injections should be given in the abdomen, so I decided to try it there. I found it was much easier to do and didn't hurt as much, since there was more skin to get a hold of. I wrote Dr. Lapraz to find out if this was okay, and he said that it was.

Three weeks after starting Xeloda, I had a blood test, which showed no reduction in my tumor markers. I was worried that Xeloda was not working, but Dr. Woliver didn't want to give up on it yet. I started a second series of the tablets and we scheduled another blood test for three weeks later. This time the results showed a reduction in my tumor markers and Dr. Woliver felt we might be on to something. I had found that with the build-up of toxins in my system, the week off of Xeloda was very difficult. I experienced lots of loose bowels and some stomachaches—not too bad, but fairly unpleasant. Still, I felt the side effects were manageable and I wanted to continue to allow the Xeloda to work.

We decided that my next appointment with Dr. Woliver would be after I returned from my second trip to Paris in the middle of May. Just before that appointment we would also schedule an abdominal CT scan to see if there were any changes in my liver, since it would have been three months since my previous scan.

Around this time, my father-in-law was hospitalized in St. Joseph, Missouri. I went back to help out since Michael was very busy at the office. The hardest thing was taking all of my medicines with me—they took up almost an entire suitcase of their own! I was extremely close to my in-laws, Esther and Lou. They were the "salt of the earth" and I loved them dearly. I was shocked to see that both of them had lost a great deal of weight since the last time I had seen them. It was very important for me to be there to drive Esther back and forth to the hospital and get her to eat some food to build up her strength. At that time, Lou was 89 and Esther was 84, and they were still living on their own in the house where Michael grew up. St. Joseph is a beautiful town, and their neighborhood had wonderful tree-lined streets. I'm always impressed with how green everything is in Missouri.

Esther had arranged for a car to pick me up at the Kansas City Airport, which was a 30-minute drive from St. Joseph. I had the driver drop me off at the hospital. Upon my arrival, I found that a bone marrow biopsy had been scheduled for my father-in-law that afternoon. I was very concerned that they would be putting an 89 year-old man in poor health through such a difficult procedure, but I was told that because of an irregular blood test they thought it was necessary in order to rule out cancer. Lou had already signed the form authorizing the test, and he got through it like the trooper he was, but Esther was quite upset at the possibility that he may have cancer. I spoke with the oncologist there and made an appointment for when the results would be back. Lou was soon feeling much better. He was discharged a couple of days later and we brought him home. The day after he got home, we went to see the oncologist and the news was great—no cancer. It was like a cloud had lifted from over both of them. I explained to the oncologist that I didn't want Lou going through another bone marrow biopsy at his age. I also told him I had discussed it with Lou's urologist and that he had concurred with me. Unfortunately, a year later the oncologist went right ahead and did another one as a follow up. Again it was negative. I could see these tests were very difficult on Lou and emotionally upsetting for both of them.

Many people do not question what tests have been ordered for them or learn about what alternatives might exist. This may or may not have been a necessary test, but age should have been a consideration. The second bone marrow biopsy was done when Lou was 90 years old, and still in poor health. Michael and I tried to get to Missouri every couple of months for a visit. I knew that my cancer was a huge concern for them and it was important that they see for themselves that I really was okay. Having advanced cancer helps one understand why people in their 80s or 90s are concerned about how much time they have left and what the quality of that time will be. Esther, Lou and I always encouraged each other to make plans for future times together. This was important for all of us—having something to look forward to. (Since I wrote this chapter, sadly, Lou passed away from heart failure at age 91. Esther had a severe stroke, which left her bed-ridden and unable to speak. She lived in a nursing home near Michael's brother, Alan, until she passed away in 2005.)

After I returned from Missouri, my stepson, David, started getting his college acceptances. He hit the big time, being accepted to Harvard, Yale, Amherst, the Huntsman Program at Penn, John Hopkins, Georgetown and Trinity. Wow—how impressed was I? Now he had to make the difficult decision of where to go. He settled on Yale, which was his favorite when he had visited college campuses the year before. I was very excited about his decision for I thought it offered the most well rounded education of all of them. But really, how could he have gone wrong! I thought back about my own college decision and remembered that I had had no choice about where to go. We were poor and I had to work my way through college, taking a full course load while working 40 hours a week. So it was the local university for me. Fortunately, that happened to be the University of Arizona, and I had a wonderful experience there. Today I'm still an avid Wildcat's fan—especially during basketball season!

Another thing I had to look forward to was attending David's college graduation. To be honest, at that time, I did stress about the fact that I might not be around to see him graduate. But I was able to let go of the fear and focused on attending the first Parent's Weekend, which was just a month after classes began. For me it was important to acknowledge that I did have the fear, to feel it, and then move beyond it. There were times that people would tell me that I should never have negative thoughts, that there should only be positive thoughts in my head. That might be a nice ideal, but I believe it's totally unrealistic. I would worry more about someone who can't get their emotions out so that they can deal with them.

Three months had passed since our first trip to Paris and it was time to go again. This was to be a "twin trip" since both Michael and Len were unable to get away. We would be there in May when the weather is wonderful, but we wouldn't have the luxury of a built-in translator since Kim had already moved back to the States, and was then living in San Francisco.

As soon as we arrived in Paris we took a cab to the lab and, to our surprise, found that it was closed. I was dismayed because I had emailed the owner of the lab from the States and he had confirmed our appointments for that day. We were concerned that the results might not get to Dr. Lapraz in time for him to order our prescriptions. We called Dr. Lapraz to make sure he was going to be at his office for our appointment. He answered the phone and said he was very surprised that the lab was closed because it was the day before a national holiday. This meant it would be two days before we could get our blood drawn. He said he would speak with the lab about putting a rush on the results so he could have them in time. He also said he would alert the pharmacy that we would be coming in with the prescription on Friday and would need to pick up the medicines that evening or early the next morning since our flight home was at noon on Saturday.

At our appointment with Dr. Lapraz, he asked how I was doing and if I had been able to stay on the scheduled medicines. I understood why this was an important question. I had a lot of medicines to take, and they didn't taste good. But Dr Lapraz bases his treatment on how well the medicines are working. If a patient didn't take the medicines diligently, he might feel he needed to alter the course of the treatment when, in reality, if they had been taken as scheduled, the results could show that they were working. We made another appointment for Friday, when he felt he would have received the blood test results. Each time I see Dr. Lapraz, I get a real lift—he is so warm and caring.

Cheryl and I left his office feeling great. Once again, we had several days to enjoy Paris before we had our next appointment. It was a gorgeous day and we spent the afternoon walking along the Rue de Rivoli and visiting The Tuileries Gardens. It was very crowded around the pond—many Parisians were basking in the warm sun. As we had learned from our experience at the lab, many businesses had closed to take advantage of a four-day weekend. But, stores were open, so we walked to the Champs Elysées and went shopping!

The next morning, I awoke feeling sick to my stomach. I wondered at the time if it was something I ate. (I know now that the timing was right for stomach pains caused by the build up in my system of toxins from taking Xeloda.) So, Cheryl and I spent the day in our hotel room watching CNN and the BBC (since they were the only television channels in English), playing cards and ordering room service. We had fun just being together, since we don't get the chance to see each other as often as we would like. Cheryl brought her laptop to work on some reports which we also used to email our husbands and check on what was happening at our offices.

On Wednesday, the lab was finally open. We went there first thing and explained how important it was to get the results to Dr. Lapraz by Friday. They told us that Dr. Lapraz had already spoken with them. They didn't speak English, and we didn't speak French, but somehow we understood each other. Cheryl and I had taken two years of French in college over 30 years ago and some of it comes back each trip.

We remembered how to get to the great café near the lab. We ate breakfast, walked to the Arc de Triomphe and down the Champs Elysées, where we found some adorable clothes for Cheryl's grandson, Noah. Paris is a wonderful diversion from all of the medical stuff! If you have to go to a city out of the States for medical reasons, you couldn't pick a more beautiful spot.

Our Friday appointment was full of good news. Dr. Lapraz felt that I had improved and that my body showed signs of combating the cancer. As before, Cheryl had also gotten a blood test. In looking over her report, he questioned her about which vitamins and antioxidants she was taking. She was very proud of the dietary supplements she'd been taking and proceeded to mention them all. Dr. Lapraz then told her that her body was over-saturated with antioxidants and that she should go off them immediately. He told her that he was prescribing medicines that would get her into balance. Antioxidants theoretically are a good thing, but too sharp an increase in their consumption over a long period of time can have an adverse reaction. That same risk of an adverse reaction exists for any drug that is overused—particularly for synthetic drugs, which have a much higher concentration of active ingredients than the plants they were originally derived from. Adverse drug reactions (ADR) were the fourth leading cause of death in American hospitals in 1997, behind heart disease, cancer and vascular disease, according to a study of 39 U.S. hospitals published in JAMA, April 15, 1998.

This really made me think about all the books people read telling them to take certain vitamins and antioxidants in order to prevent cancer. Without performing a blood test on every reader, how can the author possibly know that the combination they are touting is good for everyone who reads their book? For example, since my cancer has metastasized, I have learned that oncologists don't want patients taking antioxidants during chemotherapy. The chemo is trying to kill cancer cells, while antioxidants work to protect cells. I'm not saying that antioxidants and vitamins aren't good. It's more about knowing which supplements, and what dosage of them is good for each individual person.

Dr. Lapraz also told me that my tumor markers (CA15-3) were down, and that the levels of estrogen in my system were also reduced. He said that my resistance to the aggression of the cancer was starting to get organized. We ended the appointment with hugs and a promise that I would return in early November.

Cheryl and I hurried off to the pharmacy with our prescriptions in hand. The people at the pharmacy were very concerned because Dr. Lapraz had told them that we would be there a couple of hours earlier. Now they felt they might not be able to get the prescriptions filled before we needed to leave. Dr. Lapraz is so thorough with all of his patients that he's always running behind. I never mind sitting an extra hour or so in his waiting room because I know that when I'm in his office, he will be spending as long as it takes with me, and not worrying about time. We always bring a book to the office because, naturally, all the magazines in his waiting room are in French. I've never seen anyone there upset because of the wait.

We agreed that we would be at the pharmacy the next morning when they opened, and they said they would have everything ready. There would be many more bottles and tablets to take back this time because I would be bringing home a six-month supply. Saturday morning we took a cab to the pharmacy, then rushed back to the hotel and barely had time to pack the medicines in our suitcases before leaving for our noon flight. Cheryl and I both were exhausted, and were very relieved by the time we slid into our seats and headed home.

Back in Santa Barbara, I had a blood test and CT scan on the Monday following our flight home from Paris. I was scheduled to see Dr. Woliver on Wednesday to go over the results. My tumor markers were down to 45.3 (normal range being 0-31.3 at the Santa Barbara lab), which was even lower than it had been the week before in Paris, when they were 60.9 (normal range at the Paris lab was 0-28). But, the most important thing was that for the first time, the CT scan showed a reduction in the size of the main tumor in my liver. It went from 3 cm to 1.2 cm in diameter. The tumor in my spleen went from 2 cm to 1.75cm in diameter. Dr. Woliver had always thought that the lesion in my spleen wasn't cancer, but now questioned if it was. This was the first time that the radiologist's report had said that there was a significant change. When I told Dr. Woliver I thought the results were due to a combination of Xeloda and the plant-based medicines, he said he wasn't going to knock the plant-based medicines with results like this! Michael and I just floated out of his office; we were on such a high. There was a real reason to celebrate that night!

Our June lab work showed that the tumor markers had continued to fall to 36.2. The combination was still working! I routinely had some diarrhea and stomach upset the day after going off Xeloda, but nothing else. It was tolerable.

June marked David's high school graduation. It was so exciting to watch him give his speech as the president of the student body. He might even have a career in politics! He received so many awards.

Then it was July and time for me to write a personal letter to the people who sponsored me for the Avon 3-Day Walk the previous year. I wanted to explain how new research had helped me over the last year. It was important for them to know that money raised for research really does help. I asked them to sponsor me again for the walk that coming October. Within a week of sending the letters I had met my minimum pledge requirement. Next I needed to get in some training walks!

The economy had been taking a beating all throughout 2001. But that generally didn't effect my greeting card company too much. Usually, when money is tight, people buy more greeting cards instead of purchasing gifts. The greeting card industry has always been thought of as relatively recession proof. But this time the poor economy was hurting most of the people I knew in the industry.

One thing in particular drove the matter home. For the previous four years we had received a large order for holiday cards from Sears. But this year the buyer told me she had to cut holiday orders by 40% and was told to buy from only one vendor. That meant no order for us. She said she was sorry and that she felt we had the best ethnic cards she had seen. It bothered her that she couldn't give us a holiday order. We had called on her at her office in Chicago a few months before, and she had indicated then that she was going to place an even larger order than the year before. We were shocked to hear there would be no order from Sears that year.

This created a great deal of stress at the office. I tried explaining to my staff that we really didn't want one account to be so important, and that we would need to get several smaller ones to make up the difference. I knew that stress wasn't good for me. Dr. Lapraz had been worried about the levels of stress I was under. A study published by Swedish researchers in 2003 followed approximately 1,500 women for 24 years. It found that those who had significant stress in the five years before the study had twice the risk for developing breast cancer as women who did not. This study was interesting to read, and it gave substance to what I had been told on numerous occasions—that stress can be very detrimental to one's health.

At the end of August I received an email from Dr. Woliver about my latest CT scan and blood work-up. He has always been so wonderful about informing me of my test results as soon as he gets them. We usually correspond through email. This one was a cute email. He wrote: "The scan looks good! The lesions are stable to slightly improved. No new lesions. Xeloda is working, perhaps with a little help from its friends from France." My tumor markers showed another improvement to 31.8— almost in normal range of 31.3 and lower. So all was going very well healthwise. I immediately emailed Dr. Lapraz with the results, and he was thrilled.

"Self-help must precede help from others. Even for making certain of help from heaven, one has to help oneself."

—MORARJI R. DESAI, FORMER PRIME MINISTER OF INDIA

CHAPTER SEVEN

Terrorist Attacks and Stress at Work

I will never forget the morning of September 11, 2001. My twin sister called and told me to turn on the television. An airplane had crashed into one of the twin towers of the World Trade Center. I became glued to the set and then saw the second plane crash into the other tower. My tears just flowed. We soon learned about the third plane that dove into the Pentagon and the fourth plane that went down in a field near Pittsburgh. So many lives taken by so many senseless acts of terrorism—I was very sad.

I suddenly remembered that my greeting card company sold cards to stores in both the World Trade Center and the Pentagon. I worried about the people that I had spoken with on the telephone so many times. Something like this affects everyone—not just those who live in the vicinity. My company also produced greeting cards for the Wildlife Conservation Society (WCS), which is headquartered at the Bronx Zoo in New York. I called to see how they were handling what had taken place. I discovered that the brother of one of the WCS photographers had died in the attack. She watched the plane hit the building from her apartment and knew that her brother was probably at work in the building. How could anyone ever get over that vision? It was so hard for me to let go of the image, how would this woman ever be able to look out her window again without seeing that tragedy unfold before her.

The events of that day created a great deal of emotional and financial stress at our office. Suddenly orders were being cancelled by stores in New York and Washington D.C. Many stores located around the World Trade Center simply closed down and had no idea when they would reopen. It was a difficult time.

A few days later, we received a beautiful painting from one of our artists, along with a note saying she felt a need to paint something meaningful after all of the tragedy. Painting was like therapy for her. This painting depicted children from all nations holding onto a flagpole from which the United States flag was unfurled. Her message for the card was, "*All we want for the holidays is love and peace.*" We felt this image was so important, that we did a special printing of the card, and made a donation to a 9/11 disaster relief fund from the proceeds. The Los Angeles Times even showed the image in an article about holiday cards that were patriotic or carried a message of unity. I think most Americans wanted to do something to help those who suffered from the attacks. This was what we were able to do.

Unfortunately, anthrax attacks were next on the agenda. It was so horrible. People were afraid to send mail because it could result in a family member or friend contracting a deadly disease. This had a huge effect on the greeting card industry. The holidays were right around the corner, and because of the fear of anthrax, people did not buy or send holiday cards. This meant that the stores that had purchased our cards returned them after the holidays. It was an enormous problem for a small company like ours. I understood why people didn't want to send cards and I definitely didn't blame them. Nevertheless—more stress!

I felt so terrible about what was going on in the world, but I did get some good personal news. My tumor markers were within the normal range—at 31.1. This was the first time they had been in the normal range, and I was thrilled. I was also told that most of my liver enzyme levels were also in the normal range. That meant that the combination of Xeloda and the plant-based medicines were continuing to work for me.

In October, Michael and I flew to New York and rented a car to drive to Connecticut for parent's weekend during David's freshmen year at Yale. It was just one month after the 9/11 attacks and we wondered how airline travel would be. It really wasn't too bad. Before going to Connecticut, we stopped at the Bronx Zoo to meet with the Wildlife Conservation Society. We spent several hours looking through thousands of slides and photographs, picking new images for the next set of cards we would be producing. Then we took off for New Haven. This was the first time I had seen Yale, and it was all that Michael and David had told me. The campus was a dream to me. Who in the world wouldn't have wanted to go to this incredible university?

Shortly after we returned home, it was time for our third trip to Paris. This time, Cheryl and Len couldn't go, so it would be a romantic getaway for just Michael and me. We planned to make it more like a vacation than a medical trip. We decided to stay at the same hotel as on our first trip. Its location was central to both the lab and Dr. Lapraz's office, plus we were already familiar with taking the metro to and from the hotel.

Going to the lab for the blood test became routine. Our first visit with Dr. Lapraz was very comforting. But we were quite anxious for the next appointment when all the blood results would be back. We wanted to know how the medicines were working. The wonderful thing about having to wait for the results was that we got to spend time exploring Paris!

It was early November, and I learned that Paris is beautiful no matter what time of year it is. We discovered a park we hadn't been to before.

Walking through it, holding hands, with a nice crisp fall breeze in the air, we felt as though we were Parisian. We saw some elderly couples also walking along holding hands. It was like a scene out of a movie. When I think about Paris, these are the moments I like to reflect on—the times between lab visits and doctor appointments.

At our second appointment with Dr. Lapraz, we found that my tumor markers were indeed down and that many of the indices he was following had improved. But many other indices had actually gone up considerably because of the extreme stress I had been under at work. All this negative activity had put me at risk.

I could see that Dr. Lapraz was worried for me. We discussed the stress at my office, and he said I needed to make some choices because my health was being compromised. He explained that the blood tests showed my body was trying to fight the cancer, but that the stress was counteracting the good that was being done. I knew I needed to do something to lower the stress. I also knew that the only way I was really going to be able to do that was to either sell the company or get an investor who could come in and run it. As we prepared to leave his office, Dr. Lapraz told me that his own stress would be increased because of his worry for me. He said I needed to let him know as soon as I did something to lower my level of stress.

Because of his worry about my health, Dr. Lapraz prescribed even more medicines than he had previously. There were so many bottles and tablets that we had to buy another suitcase just to hold them all! On the plane ride back, Michael and I talked about the stress and about how it was affecting my health. I decided to start working on selling the company. That was a very difficult thing for me to do. In many ways, I think I identified my existence through my company, which I'm sure was not very healthy. I'm also sure it's why everything associated with the company affected me on such a personal level. I watched Michael run his company, and he handled it very differently. For him, it was just a business—important, but not his personal mission in life. However, I didn't think I would be able to distance myself from everything that was going on at my company. Michael suggested that we just close the doors of the greeting card company—that my life was far more important.

Around this time, I received a call from a friend in the greeting card industry about a joint effort we had been working on. I told him about what the doctor said regarding lowering stress in my life. He said that perhaps we should consider putting together a deal for his company to distribute our cards. Michael and I thought it was something to check out. Since our anniversary was right around the corner, we decided to fly to Seattle, celebrate our anniversary and meet with my friend in person. During this trip, I was feeling a lot of pain in my stomach, and couldn't help but wonder if it was the cancer spreading. I could barely stay focused on what was being said in the meetings. I was thankful that Michael was there and could take over for me. We thought that my friend's company was great, but in order to make a deal with them work, we felt I would still have had to be much too involved in day-to-day operations.

While we were in Seattle, Dr. Woliver left a message at our hotel saying that the results of my latest blood tests were all very good. He thought the pain I had been experiencing was caused by a build-up of toxins from taking Xeloda. So I took a three-week vacation from Xeloda in order to allow my body to recover. At our next appointment, Dr. Woliver decided to try a new regimen of two weeks on Xeloda, and two weeks off—while staying with the same dosage. That really did help.

In January, 2002 I met with my staff and told them I needed to make some changes to lower my stress. I explained that my doctor was very concerned about my health. At that time, a venture capital firm had shown some interest in investing in the company, and I told my staff about it. I hoped that something like this would allow me to take more of a back seat in the operation.

We decided that for the present, we would try to take care of the needs of our customers, but we wouldn't create a new catalog. One of the responsibilities I attended to personally was the production of all our catalogs and preparing the cards for printing. This was exactly the kind of stress I needed to avoid. We would simply send out our existing catalog when people needed one. We also decided to pare our collection of cards down to only the bestsellers. Over the previous two years, since my cancer had metastasized, I had allowed our collections to become too big. Because I was so preoccupied by my disease, all we had done was add new cards, while not eliminating poor sellers. During that meeting with my staff there were a lot of tears, but they understood I didn't have a choice in the matter. I told them I would keep them informed of whatever happened.

I also had a meeting with my banker. The events surrounding 9/11 had put us under severe financial pressure. She told me she thought that my company could qualify for one of the low interest Small Business Administration loans that were being given to businesses hurt by the 9/11 disasters. When I looked into it, the SBA said that we hadn't been hurt enough from the actual events of 9/11. Since we had been affected by the resulting downturn in the economy and the anthrax scare, the loan program did not apply to us.

When I look back, I realize that I just wasn't sure what to do with the company. I could try to get an investor to help me to hire someone to take over some of my responsibilities, or I could try to get a loan to do the same thing, or, I could just try to sell it. I was worried about the stress and how it was affecting my ability to fight the cancer. Yet, this was still a very emotional move for me. It was like letting go of a child. I had many employees and many artists that were very dear to me. I wanted to take care of them. I had a great deal of trouble sleeping at night.

This was also a difficult time for Michael. He knew how hard this all was for me and he was worried about my health. We had many discussions about it, and finally decided that the investor idea wasn't a good one. Most investors seemed interested in absurdly high rates of return, and we were just small potatoes to them. We decided that the best course of action was to either sell the company or just close it down. One option was to declare bankruptcy and close the doors, but I didn't really want to do that. We decided to take out a second mortgage on our home and pay off the debt that the company had accumulated. It was a difficult time to be trying to sell a business. Michael was amazing through the whole thing. He was very willing to go into debt in order to relieve the stress in my life. He assured me that we would get through it. How do you ever pay that back? Whenever I brought it up, Michael's response was, "It's just money." Being confronted with these issues brought new meaning to those words that I had heard so many times. Having cancer has definitely helped me realize what really counts in life.

The good news was that my cancer was now stable. I was not in remission, but stable. Still, I knew that I was skating on thin ice because I remained under a tremendous amount of stress. If I was going to be able to reduce the stress permanently and remain stable, something would have to happen sooner rather than later.

When people meet me and learn about my cancer, they often ask if my cancer is in remission. I explain that, as I understand it, remission is when cancer is undetectable in the body. My cancer can still be found throughout my liver, but it's not active. I believe that being stable is the answer for me. My aim is to keep the cancer contained and my body healthy so that it won't produce any new tumors.

May, 2002 came and off to Paris we went. Michael and I were excited because Cheryl and Len were traveling with us. We wanted to take Len to all of the places we had discovered, and we have so much fun being together. This would also be Len's first meeting with Dr. Lapraz. We dropped our luggage at the hotel and took the metro to the lab. Len would see the routine we had experienced on our previous trips. After the lab, we had our first appointment with Dr. Lapraz. After we had all spoken for a while in his office, Cheryl and Len went in to the waiting room while I had my physical examination and then we reversed it so Cheryl could have her physical. It was so nice seeing Dr. Lapraz again, and Len was quite impressed with him. It was also fun to be back in Paris, and there was no better time than the spring! We spent three days taking in the sights.

Then it was time to see Dr. Lapraz for our second appointment, where we would go over the results of the blood work. The test results showed that I was still under too much stress. Although some of the indices that Dr. Lapraz followed had improved a bit since I had made the decision to sell my company, the stress was still taking a huge toll on my body. My tumor markers were down to 24, but my estrogen level was up. I still had a lot of work to do in order to lower the stress and enable my body to fight the cancer.

I was fascinated when I heard Dr. Lapraz going over Cheryl's blood test results. He asked her if she had only taken her medicines for three months instead of six. She said yes, that she had misplaced them when they moved to a new home and had only recently located them while unpacking. He knew that the blood work didn't look like it would have if she had been on the medicines for the full six months. Dr. Lapraz faxed our new prescriptions to the pharmacy. When we said our goodbyes, he said he hoped my company would soon be sold so my stress level would go down. He told me to remain positive always.

After our meeting with Dr. Lapraz, Len wanted to see the Picasso Museum. We hadn't been there before and we enjoyed it very much. Afterwards we stopped into a great little art gallery where Cheryl and Len bought a painting by a Russian artist. Another thing that we hadn't done on previous trips was to take a boat trip along the Seine River. The weather was perfect so we climbed aboard and enjoyed seeing Paris from the river.

Len had to leave Paris a few days early for a legal conference in Chicago. After he left, Cheryl, Michael and I went to London for the day, taking a bullet train through the Chunnel. It was such a great day. The Queen's Jubilee was going to be taking place the following week and the whole city had been decorated for the celebrations. We went to Buckingham Palace, saw the changing of the guard, and all the rehearsals for the Jubilee. It was so much fun. We shopped until we dropped and then took the late train back to Paris, relaxing over dinner and a nice glass of Bordeaux.

After that trip, I came back to Santa Barbara with a strong resolve to finally do what needed to be done regarding my company. My health was just too important to string it out any longer.

We decided to close down operations as of September 30, 2002. We made the decision at the beginning of June, so we had four full months to wind everything down. I told my staff that we were still working on selling the company, and that I hoped someone would want to keep it intact, but if that didn't happen I needed to just close the doors. We told our sales representatives what was going on and that we would only take orders until July 15th. We also sent a letter to all of our artists explaining everything, and to say that we hoped to be able to sell the company. I also told them that if we didn't, I would refer each of them to a greeting card company I thought would be a good match for them.

In a letter to our customers, we announced a going-out-of-business sale for the month of August. We also sent a press release to trade journals and the general media. I was amazed at the immediate response. Our local newspaper called and sent a photographer to do a story about my selling the company, and about my cancer. Then every single trade journal for the greeting card industry published our press release. Some even put it up on their web site the day they received it. Calls started to pour in from local people and other greeting card companies expressing interest in buying the company. I also got calls from many people I knew in the industry. They told me how sorry they were about my cancer and wanted me to know they would help in any way they could. I was so very touched.

But, what moved me most were the letters I received from my artists. I never knew just how much publishing their art had meant to them, and how it had changed many of their lives. I cried as I read each heartfelt story. This was why I had gone into business in the first place—to publish affordable art, not just a card to read and throw away, but something that was good enough to be framed and kept. I wanted to provide a way for artists to get their art seen and appreciated. One letter in particular said it all:

Dear Carol:

Last night I returned from Guatemala. This morning I opened your package. I have tears running down my cheeks, not for me but for you. I know how hard you have worked for this company. Although I do not "know you," I do know you very well. You have been everything to me as an artist and a person.

Because you are leaving this chapter of your life, I want to tell you what your encouragement has given me.

My history, to make a long story short, started by supporting myself and my child at the age of 16. Because of those circumstances I worked jobs that I could get, and never the jobs that I liked. I worked for years and years in laboratories, but painted every night. My identity was shallow and I did art to express my feelings, my hopes, and what I saw in others.

One day a friend picked up one of your cards and encouraged me to send my art to you. I did it just to satisfy her. I never dreamed I would hear from you! You not only responded in person but showed interest and enthusiasm in my work, so I kept painting.

When the first cards came out, I showed them to my friends and family. They saw with new eyes what they had seen for years and said, "Wow! You are really a good artist!" I became proud, and I kept painting.

I left the laboratories, where I worked with nitroglycerin and rocket propellant, and other things that go BOOM in the night. I returned to school. I majored in graphic arts and started working for the Salt Lake Newspaper in the art department, where I worked for six years. Last fall (Sept. 6th) I quit to pursue work as a full time artist.

As I mentioned, I just returned from a trip to Guatemala, where poverty is terrible and living conditions are hard. I want to spread the vision of their plight. Naturally, there was lots of subject material! When I opened my mail at home I found two potential offers from publishers of children's books. One about poverty and one about the strength of one woman saving many children during the Holocaust. True stories. Can you believe it?

I do not know where all this will lead, but I do know that my sense of identity and self worth are directly attributed to you and your faith in others. I do know I want to also get the word of peace out. I do know that people like us can change the world one glance at a time...and we have the chutzpah to do it!

In addition to giving me the courage to develop myself, you have given me peace of mind and hope in my sister, Carrie's, ovarian cancer. I love her so much and it frightens me to lose her. I see through you that life and cancer are a process that we live each day. I have discovered through my relationship with you, that in your soul, I see my own identity. Carol, thank you from the bottom of my heart.

I hope I will still be able to reach you by email and that we can chat from time to time. You have become a part of me. Good luck and good health and G-d's speed.

Fondly, Suzanne Tornquist

I promptly cried! Closing down the business was difficult. Reading letters like this was of great importance to me—it kept me going.

In 2003 I had the opportunity to finally meet Suzanne Tornquist. It was such a thrill to give her a big hug and let her know in person just how much her letter of thanks had meant to me. Many times we want to express how we feel, but our lives become so hectic that time passes and the opportunity escapes us.

All of the local people who had expressed interest in buying my company were very nice, but none of them knew anything about the greeting card industry and most would have wanted me to stay involved. I realized that this would have meant even more stress. I would have been working hard to educate them about the industry and trying to help them be successful in a very difficult business. That was totally out of the question. I also spoke with several large greeting card companies, but none of them were a good match for us.

Then on August 19, 2002, I got a call from Dale Byars, the owner of a company named Caravan International. He had heard about my cancer and knew that I was planning to close the company. He asked if I would be interested in selling it to him. I knew all about Caravan. They produced wonderful Asian greeting cards. Since my company also sold Asian cards, we had heard of them through sales representatives, and had seen their exhibits at trade shows. Dale was the new owner of Caravan. I hadn't heard that he had purchased Caravan from its original owners a few years before. At times like this I realized how out of touch I had become since my efforts had been split between fighting cancer and running my company.

Dale and I must have spent more than an hour on the phone that day, just talking and getting to know one another. I knew, by the end of the call, that this was the person I wanted to sell my company to. I felt not only that we were a perfect fit, but that I could trust Dale. His values were the same as mine, and he assured me he would honor all of my artists' contracts. That had been a major concern of mine. I faxed him a non-disclosure agreement, which he signed and faxed right back. Then I sent him a confidential offering that we had prepared for people who were interested in purchasing the company.

Over the next several weeks Dale and I spoke many times. Essentially we agreed to agree on all points regarding the purchase. When something is right, everything seems to fit into place. That's how this sale was. We knew that combining the two companies could make one very strong company. All of our different collections complemented each other. We never had one disagreement regarding the purchase. We both wanted it to work out, and there was give and take on each side.

At this time, as I was negotiating the sale of the company and packing everything up, I received a call telling me I had been nominated for Santa Barbara Woman Entrepreneur of the Year, an award given by a group called Women's Economic Ventures. I told them that I didn't feel qualified because I was selling my company. They said that didn't matter—that it was about what I had done since starting the company. They asked me to fax them my resume, as the committee would be meeting that evening to decide the winner. They said the person who nominated me hadn't given them many details. I had no idea who had nominated me, but figured it must have been my banker, since she was very involved with this organization.

I was in the middle of the sale, and there was so much on my plate. I really didn't have time to think about what to send them. Most things were already packed, but I found an old resume that I updated and faxed to the person who had called. Several weeks later, after attending the luncheon honoring the nominees and the winner, I realized it was an honor to have been nominated. Cheryl flew to Santa Barbara to share in the celebration. All of the women were so accomplished, I felt great to be recognized along with them.

A slight problem came up regarding the timing of the sale of the company. Dale had hoped to take a little more time to finalize things so that he could get a larger warehouse. But I was determined to close the doors of my office on September 30th. That was just a few weeks away. We had already given notice to the landlord, and because of my illness, they had allowed me to break my lease. They had already rented the space to a new tenant who was planning to move in on October first.

I definitely didn't want to have the expense of moving the inventory to a warehouse while we waited for the deal to close. I also didn't want to pay another month's rent and make the new tenants delay their move. I knew of another greeting card company that would buy my entire inventory. They were my backup if the deal with Dale fell through. I hired extra staff to box up everything in the warehouse—but we didn't know if it would be going to Caravan or to the other company. Either way, I knew it would be leaving our warehouse on September 30th.

By this time all my employees had either taken new jobs, or were staying just to help me close down the operation. None of them wanted to relocate to Texas where Caravan was headquartered. The negotiations continued, and finally Dale found a place for the inventory to be shipped. He overnighted a deposit that arrived on Friday, September 27th. The following Monday, September 30th, more than a million cards, a counting machine, and hundreds of feet of shelving left for Texas. The load filled two large trucks.

Everything just seemed to fall into place. The new tenant in our warehouse was so nice. He said he would love to have anything I didn't feel like moving out. He also needed to hire a shipping manager, and ended up hiring my shipping manager, Joyce. This was fortunate for me, because Joyce watched for mail that didn't get forwarded, and then made sure I got it. The new tenant went so far as to put in his lease that he was taking the space in "as is" condition. That meant I would get all of my damage deposit back. How lucky was I?

He knew about my cancer and I think was trying to help me out. Regardless of what he had said, I still arranged for a cleaning crew to come in after the movers left and get the place in good order. Then I put the keys in an envelope and slid it through the property manager's mail slot. As I watched that envelope disappear, I could feel the stress start to melt away!

"Fear cannot be without hope nor hope without fear."

—BENEDICT SPINOZA

CHAPTER EIGHT

Letting Go of the Fear

About two weeks before the move, Michael and I had found a great little office for me just three minutes from our house. I needed some sort of an office to finalize everything for the sale of the company. I had also agreed to create several catalogs for the new owners combining all of our products. I knew my decision to sell my company had been the right one as soon as I spent the first day in my new office. I had gone from 6,500 square feet with five full-time employees (during busy periods it had gone up to 12), 75 artists, and 80 sales representatives to a mere 200 square feet. There was just me, my computer, a fax machine, and a telephone. No stress at all!

My son, Michael, sent me a gorgeous bouquet of flowers to celebrate the sale of my company and the start of a new phase of my life with much less stress. He had been so worried about me. Naturally, I emailed Dr. Lapraz to tell him about the sale. He was so happy and, I am sure, quite relieved. He ended his reply to me with notes of encouragement, saying that he couldn't wait to see us at our next appointment in Paris.

But before our trip to Paris, it was time for my regular three-month check-up with Dr. Woliver. This time, for some reason that we couldn't quite put our finger on, Michael and I were both worried about what we would hear at this appointment. There really wasn't anything to substantiate the worry. It just seemed that after so many appointments with only good news, this might be the time for the other shoe to drop. We were always prepared to hear that my tumor markers were going up, which would mean that Xeloda had stopped working. But, once again, Dr. Woliver had only good news for us—everything looked great on the blood tests. I knew then that this type of worry would always be a part of my life. It's something I have to deal with and I'm okay with it.

We arrived in Paris on October 31, 2002. It was for my fifth trip to see Dr. Lapraz. We were surprised to see Halloween decorations in many of the shop windows—not a big deal, but they were there. Again, both Cheryl and Len were accompanying Michael and me. We had decided to try a charming little French hotel—La Régence Etoile. It was just a block from the Arc de Triomphe, and near the Champs Elysées, the fabulous boulevard where we loved to stroll during our visits.

The lab where my blood work was done was only a short walk from the hotel. After checking in we went directly to the lab. The people there remembered us, and everything went smoothly. It was Thursday, and they said they hoped to have the results for Dr. Lapraz by Monday. But they reminded us that Friday was a holiday, so the results might be delayed. From the lab, we went straight to our appointment with Dr. Lapraz. Even though it was still early in the day, patients were already backed up in his waiting room. He came out to greet us and asked if we could return at five that evening. We had no problem with that since we were all quite hungry, so we found a restaurant, had lunch, and then went back to the hotel to unpack.

That evening, during my physical exam at Dr. Lapraz's office, I noticed that it didn't hurt the way it had previously when he pressed on certain parts of my body. When I mentioned this to him, he said it was because I was finally getting into balance. I had brought him the results of the most recent blood tests that had been performed in the United States, and he was very pleased with them. Our next appointment with Dr. Lapraz was scheduled for Monday afternoon, but the lab work done in Paris ended up not coming back in time, so the appointment was changed to Wednesday.

We passed the time by sightseeing and shopping. We decided to stop by the small art gallery where Cheryl and Len had purchased a painting on a previous trip. They saw many new paintings by the same artist that they liked. Michael and I fell in love with and bought a small lithograph, as well as a wonderful painting by a French artist. We felt so comfortable being in Paris and there was always so much to do.

At our appointment with Dr. Lapraz on Wednesday, I was surprised to see a worried look on his face. During my physical exam a few days earlier, he had been so pleased. I was afraid that he had seen something troubling in the results of my Paris blood work—even though the tests done in Santa Barbara indicated everything was fine. I felt that Dr. Lapraz knew something more, because he always entered the results of my blood analysis into a computer model that helped him to understand the functioning of my body on a very detailed level. This sort of understanding can't be achieved by a traditional blood analysis that looks only at the levels of certain substances circulating in the bloodstream. An analysis that looks only at the levels of substances, and not how the body consumes or reacts to them, will always be limited. The detailed analysis and computerized diagnostic model employed by Dr. Lapraz yields a much fuller understanding.

Dr. Lapraz explained that, for one thing, he was concerned because this was the fall—a time of year (along with the spring) when climactic changes make our endocrine systems more vulnerable. These times of vulnerability are when the reoccurrence of disease often takes place, because the body is less able to fight it off. I was told that that my stress levels—although still lower than they had been one year earlier—were double what they had been six months ago. Dr. Lapraz said he was afraid that the accumulated stress I had been exposed to for the past 15 months had taken its toll. My blood work had shown that most of the indices were up significantly, showing that I was at risk. Nevertheless, this danger wasn't indicated by the test for tumor markers (which continued to drop to 20.5), because, as I mentioned before, it only measures the current level of a substance circulating in the blood.

But Dr. Lapraz said he realized that the sale of my company had only just been completed and that more time would be needed before we would see any significant difference in the levels of stress I was experiencing. When I reflected on what he said about this being a vulnerable time of year, I realized that there was a great deal of truth in it. The lump in my breast had originally been discovered in November. We had also learned that the cancer metastasized in my liver in November two years later.

At the end of our four-hour appointment with Dr. Lapraz, I asked if he had seen anything else in my blood work that concerned him. He just said that he wanted me to be in better health, but that it would take several years to see all of the results. We had only been working together for 20 months. He ordered quite a few more medicines for me than on previous trips. I just hoped we would be able to get them all into our suitcases. We usually bring one mostly empty suitcase for this purpose, but this time it looked like the prescriptions might fill two of them! Thinking back, I can't help but wonder what all of this stress would have done to me if I hadn't been protected by the plant-based medicines that I had been taking.

Dr. Lapraz was also concerned about the levels of work-related stress in Cheryl's life, and he increased her medicines as well. I'm so relieved that

Cheryl is seeing Dr. Lapraz. I sleep better at night knowing that he is protecting her against cancer.

At this appointment we also discussed the book I was writing. I asked if he would give me a written explanation of endobiogénie and elaborate on how the medicines I was taking helped me to fight cancer. Along with Dr. Duraffourd, he had just published an 800-page clinical book, which was, of course, in French. He hoped to get it translated into English. He said he thought my book would be important for the average person to read. Their book had been written for medical professionals. As we left he told me that I must write every day, and that he was very anxious to see the manuscript when it was completed.

While in Paris, we had heard about an exceptional exhibit of paintings by Matisse and Picasso at the Grand Palais. It had been in London and would go on to New York as its final destination. On Thursday we went to see this amazing exhibit. I felt sorry for anyone who went to other museums to see paintings by Matisse and Picasso during that time, because they were all at this very special exhibit. What a treat!

On Friday, the day before our departure, we went to the pharmacy to pick up the medicines. The pharmacist, Dr. Patrick Meimoun, had to make a delivery near our hotel so he loaded us and our medicines into his car and gave us a ride. What a nice man. He enjoyed speaking to Americans so he could practice his English, which was very good. We have met so many wonderful people in Paris.

Several weeks after we returned from Paris, I stubbed my big toe on my left foot while running up some stairs. I thought that I must have sprained it badly, for it turned black and blue and swelled up immediately. But, after going to a podiatrist and getting it x-rayed, I found the toe was actually broken. Thinking back about what Dr. Lapraz said, I would have to agree that things do happen to me this time of year—especially in November!

Dale Byars, the owner of Caravan, flew out to meet me and sign the final papers for the sale of the company on December 12, 2002. Everything was exactly as we had agreed right from our first conversation. We both felt the sale was final, but we did have to go through a legal procedure called a bulk sale in order to meet California state requirements. It was something like going through escrow when buying a house. A search is done to make sure neither company has liens against it, and the paperwork is submitted to the State of California, which officially records it.

In the meantime, I started working on the catalogs for the new company. I had agreed to do this as part of the sale. Michael and I spent the next couple of months laying out three new catalogs. There ended up being an 80-page everyday catalog, a 32-page animals catalog, and a 48-page holiday catalog. I worked with Dale and his sister Marti, who was also working for the company. Everything came together smoothly. The bulk sale went through without any problems, and the catalogs were completed in time for the May National Stationery Show in New York. We had all decided it would be important for me to attend the Show in order to introduce artists and buyers to the new owners of the company. A notice had been sent to all of our customers announcing the sale, and asking them to come to the booth to get copies of the new catalogs when they came to the show.

While working on the catalogs, I had regular blood tests and a CT scan. Everything still showed that I had a stable disease. I felt great physically, so this was a nice confirmation that all was going along as hoped. My appointments with Dr. Woliver, which always include blood tests, are usually every three months, and I have a CT scan every six months. When the cancer was active, appointments were every three weeks, so this was a nice break.

About this time, Angela (the friend who had originally told me about Dr. Lapraz) called and asked if I would speak with a friend of hers (Colleen

Shaffer) whose breast cancer had just metastasized in the liver. She was scheduled to start Xeloda, the same drug I was on. She had heard from Angela that I had already been on Xeloda for over a year and she wanted to know how I handled it. I was more than pleased to speak with her, so Angela gave her my number. She called and we had so much to talk about.

Although Colleen had gone through chemotherapy when her breast cancer was first diagnosed, it had metastasized in her liver. Now she was going on Xeloda. I told her that my cancer had become stable after starting Xeloda, and that I had been fortunate not to have too many side effects. I also explained how my doctor had started me on a lower dose than the manufacturer recommended because side effects could be a problem. She told me it had been helpful to speak with me, and that by telling her to think of cancer as a chronic illness like diabetes, I had given her a new way to think about her disease.

Colleen called me back after her doctor's appointment. She had been put on a higher dose of Xeloda than the one I was started on. She immediately experienced some bad side effects (blisters on her hands and feet). She wasn't able to finish the two-week cycle. I told her that Dr. Woliver felt that higher doses hadn't been found to be more effective, and that she might want to ask her doctor about lowering the dose. She thought that because she was much taller than I was, that perhaps she should be on a higher dose. Finally her doctor did reduce the dose, but still not as low as mine, and she continued to have horrible side effects and was still not able to complete the cycle. Colleen's doctor kept lowering the dose to even lower than mine. She remains on a schedule of two weeks on Xeloda and one week off. The good news is that Colleen has been on Xeloda since 2002 and her cancer has stayed stable. Like me, she does complementary treatments in addition to chemotherapy. What's wonderful is watching someone like Colleen fight her disease and then go on to help others in need. She has formed a non-profit company (Circle of Hope, Inc.) that financially and emotionally assist uninsured and underinsured individuals with breast cancer who live, work or are treated in the area where she lives, Santa Clarita Valley near Los Angeles, California.

I had soon finished my work on the catalogs and sent digital files off to Dale so he could get the catalogs printed in time for the Stationery Show. This was a huge accomplishment for me. My work in the greeting card industry was now basically done.

I decided to celebrate by taking a road trip to see my son and daughter. I hadn't visited my son, Michael, since he had taken the position as an assistant district attorney in Coos Bay, Oregon. I also wanted to see my daughter, Kim, in San Francisco. Originally I had planned to also take my dog, Mattie. But, I realized she would end up spending a lot of time alone in a strange house or apartment when we went out to eat or did something else. I decided it would be better for her to stay home with Michael.

Then Cheryl told me that she wanted to go. She would fly to Santa Barbara and we would drive to San Luis Obispo and see our aunt and uncle who lived there. Then, it would be on to San Francisco where we would see Kim, and our brother Vernon and his wife Anne. The last leg would take us to Oregon to see my son Michael. Cheryl felt she could get away from her office for a week. I'm sure she also wanted to go because she was worried about me taking such a long trip alone. In any case, it turned out great. We had so much fun. I was able to have some important, in person conversations about my cancer with both of my children. It's often hard to discuss what's going on with the cancer over the telephone. Many things are best said when you can see each other's eyes. It was also important for them to see that I really was doing fine.

Shortly after the trip, I had developed a pain right around the lower ribs on the left side of my body. I was concerned, and made an appointment with Dr. Woliver. He said he thought my symptoms sounded like shingles, but shingles are almost always accompanied by a rash and I didn't have one. He decided to schedule a bone scan for the next day just to be sure that cancer hadn't returned to my ribs. He said if a rash showed up before the scan, he would cancel it. The rash didn't appear and the bone scan came back negative. We didn't know what to think. I have spoken with people who had shingles without a rash during chemo, but it's very unusual. Shingles is dormant in the body after one has had chicken pox—which I did have as a child. Various things can trigger it, and chemotherapy is one of them. Dr. Woliver ordered something for the pain, but didn't want to treat it like shingles as long as there was no rash. It was very uncomfortable and I was happy to have something for the pain, as I was leaving for the National Stationery Show in New York.

Shortly before leaving town, I received a call from a friend of mine saying that she was going to be having dinner with a doctor friend who was a specialist in treating liver cancer, and in perfecting new techniques in liver surgery. She knew all about my cancer and wanted to know if there were any questions I wanted her to ask him. My friend lived on the East Coast and thought I might like to meet this doctor while I was in New York. He was on staff at the Montefiore Medical Center in the Bronx. The whole thing sounded very intriguing, but it wouldn't be possible for me to meet him on this trip, as I was only going to be in New York for a couple of days and every minute was accounted for. She emailed me some information about the doctor, which looked impressive. I made a mental note to possibly arrange a meeting when both Michael and I would be on the East Coast during the next Parent's Weekend at Yale.

It was so great to go to the National Stationery Show because it allowed me to have closure with the process of selling my company. I took Dale, the new owner of my company, to a meeting of the Board of Directors of the Greeting Card Association. I was able to introduce him to members of the Board, and to give a farewell speech at the end of the meeting. It was hard for me to get all of the words out without falling apart. Many of these people had been friends for nearly 15 years. Several of them had sent me wonderful cards and letters when they heard about my cancer. I wanted to let them know their concern had meant a great deal to me, and I wanted to officially say goodbye.

One of the hardest parts of selling my company was knowing I would no longer be seeing my dear friends Carole and Victor Gellineau at industry trade shows. They own a terrific greeting card company called Carole Joy Creations. I will never forget a Greeting Card Association Convention in New Orleans where the three of us enjoyed a wonderful evening. This was before I met my husband, and Carole and Victor and I danced together all night long—we had so much fun! After Michael and I got married the four of us would go to dinner whenever we had the opportunity.

This time I was only going to be in New York for the first two days of the show, since Michael and I were leaving for Paris the day after I got back. I wasn't able to get together with Carole and Victor, but we hugged and said we would stay in touch—which we have. We were competitors in the greeting card industry, but that never interfered with our friendship. Carole calls to check in on a regular basis and see how I'm doing. That means more to me than I can say!

At the Stationery Show, I was glad to meet Dale's sister, Marti, after working with her so closely over the telephone. She was exactly as I had pictured—so much like her brother, with a strong Texas drawl and full of warmth. That year at the Stationery Show I felt like I was officially turning over the reigns of my company.

I was also happy to finally meet some of the artists that I had spoken with numerous times. Because of my cancer, I had missed several shows in recent years, and hadn't been able to meet them in person. Suzanne

Tornquist had come to New York from Utah just so we could finally meet. She was the artist who sent me the remarkable letter of thanks when she heard about the sale of the company (included in an earlier chapter). I couldn't wait to meet her. She came with her daughter and granddaughter. Many years earlier, I had purchased one of Suzanne's paintings. It had been used for the cover of one of our catalogs. I felt so touched by it that I asked if I could buy it. It showed two boys with their arms around each other walking down a snowy village road. A menorah can be seen through the window of one home in the background, and a Christmas wreath can be seen on a door of another. This was what my company was about—cultural diversity and understanding. Michael and I had the painting framed, and it hangs for all to see as they enter our home.

As we were packing for Paris, I started thinking how much my life had changed in such a short time. This was going to be our sixth trip to see Dr. Lapraz in two years and three months. I was learning so much about my body, and the ways that various things can affect the balance of my health. Before getting cancer, this wasn't even part of my thinking. I had been a vegetarian, not for health reasons, but out of concern regarding cruelty to animals. When my son Michael was in the eighth grade, he brought home pictures of how animals were raised for slaughter in small pens where they couldn't move. That played on my mind and I gave up eating meat. Perhaps, if I had stopped eating meat for health reasons, I would have been more aware of what chemicals could do and how foods like dairy affect the body. There is a delicate balance and throwing it off can create problems.

At the Paris airport, Cheryl, Len, Michael and I were used to getting through customs and catching a cab to our hotel without difficulty. Our routine was to check in at the hotel, drop off our luggage, and go directly to the lab for blood tests. We knew that every minute counted in making sure the results would get to Dr. Lapraz in time for our appointment. It would have been much easier if we could have gotten the lab work done in the States and brought the results with us. We could have shaved at least three days off our trip.

But, at the time, we hadn't been able to find a lab in Santa Barbara that could complete all the tests that Dr. Lapraz needed. In particular, they seemed to have problems with tests involving the breakdown of alkaline phosphatases between bones, liver and intestines. Some labs seemed to feel that if the total alkaline phosphatases were within normal range, there was no need to do the breakdown. But Dr. Lapraz needed that breakdown for his computer model. Something else that caused problems was the test for osteocalcin, a bone protein. It's an indicator of bone metabolism. The test for it requires a special extraction technique, and not all labs can do it. Fortunately, the lab I currently use in Santa Barbara can do all of the tests that are needed. Now I am able to bring the blood test results with me to Paris.

During this trip another American patient of Dr. Lapraz's, who Michael and I had met in Los Angeles, had also traveled to France. She had originally found out about him because she worked with the brother of Angela—who had first told me about Dr. Lapraz.

This patient has breast cancer as well. She had just finished chemotherapy when we saw her in Paris. She was scheduled for radiation and wanted to see Dr. Lapraz before those treatments began. She, her husband, Cheryl, Len, Michael and I all took over a great Chinese restaurant near our hotel. The food was delicious and the cook made things for us to try that weren't even on the menu. We had so much fun. This woman takes Dr. Lapraz's instructions very seriously, and has made me question my occasional consumption of dairy products. She is a good influence on me! She's the one that got me to read Dr. Jane Plant's book.

The French Open Tennis Tournament was going on while we were in Paris, and Cheryl and Len had been able to get tickets for all of us through a friend of theirs. The tickets were for opening day at Center Court. We couldn't wait and prayed for a nice sunny day. That's exactly what we got. We couldn't have chosen better weather. We got to see great tennis played by such notables as Serena Williams, Roger Federer, Amelie Mauresmo (a great French player) and one of my favorite tennis players, Andre Agassi. It was such a beautiful day. After the matches, we found an incredible restaurant. We were underdressed in our casual clothes, but they were so nice and accommodating. And the food was the best we had had in Paris—and that's saying a lot! We had worried about how the French would react to Americans because of the war in Iraq, but they were all courteous, gracious and very helpful.

My clinical exam with Dr. Lapraz went well. He agreed with Dr. Woliver that I didn't have shingles. He said that after I had broken my toe in November, I had started to walk differently and that had created a blockage on my left side. He explained the pain I had been feeling in my ribs was caused by something like pinched nerves. He arranged for another doctor in his office, an osteopath, to work on me before our next appointment, when we would go over my blood test results. It was nice to be going to a doctor who was treating my whole body. His approach was so different from most doctors I had seen in the United States. My whole body was being put in balance—not just my liver.

Cheryl and I were pleased to find we had lost about eight pounds each. I had cut out dairy and soy while limiting carbohydrates, and it was working. Of course, if our thyroids had still been shut down, then anything we tried wouldn't have worked.

Dr. Lapraz told me that everything looked very good, but noticed that I seemed worried. I told him a couple of things were on my mind. The first was that I had been given two years to live by my first oncologist. It was now three and a half years since that diagnosis. I couldn't help but wonder how much time I really had left. He said I needed to realize that I had many years left, and to let go of the fear. He assured me he would know from my exams if something were going wrong, and that he would be able to adjust my medications accordingly.

Secondly, I mentioned that I had noticed my tumor markers— while still in the normal range—had been moving upward. Naturally, that concerned me. He explained that, in his experience, fluctuations in tumor markers were typical among patients who had been on Xeloda for a long time. I hadn't heard that before, and it eased my worries. He most definitely knows what to say to quiet my brain. He also mentioned that yoga would be a good thing for me to start. It was funny he should say that, because I had just told Cheryl I wanted to get into a yoga class when I got back to Santa Barbara!

Tuesday evening we were scheduled for our final appointment with Dr. Lapraz, then we were going to go out for dinner. I hadn't been worried about what the lab results were going to be. I was feeling very calm when Dr. Lapraz gave me the good news that, actually, my tumor markers were now going down. They were at 23.3, and many of the other functions he was following were much improved.

I can't explain what this trip meant to me emotionally. I felt like a huge weight had been lifted off my shoulders. I learned that tumor markers fluctuate, and that as long as they were in normal range, I shouldn't be concerned. I had also let go of the "years left" fear. I had been able to quiet my brain.

During the appointment Dr. Lapraz mentioned that he had been invited to speak at a World Health Organization conference in Tunisia, and that he was planning to be presenting my case. That interested me very much. He told me that, for reasons of confidentiality, he wouldn't use my name, but instead refer to me by a case number. I told him I really didn't care if he used my name, and he said that maybe the next time he spoke, I could be there.

While Cheryl was going over her test results with Dr. Lapraz, I saw the osteopath. He worked on my body to loosen up the congestion on my left side and also said he was happy that I was planning to start practicing yoga. He told me that I wasn't breathing correctly. As children, girls are often times told to hold in their stomach so it will look flat. This results in shallow breathing. I learned how to breathe through my stomach on that trip. Cheryl worked with me on this, because she had previously trained patients of hers to do that during relaxation exercises.

By the time all the results were entered into Dr. Lapraz's computer program, and he had written the prescriptions and faxed them to the pharmacy, it was after 10:30 at night. But Paris stays up late, so it was no problem finding a wonderful restaurant that was open. Again, something quite different than what we are used to in Santa Barbara.

We spent the following day on a visit to Versailles. I had been there some years before, but Michael had never been there. May is the perfect time to visit, the gardens are beautiful, it's not too hot, and the tourist season hasn't really begun. There are many wonderful places to visit just outside of Paris, but the city itself is so beautiful. With so many interesting places to see, it will take many trips before we have a chance to discover them all.

We went to the pharmacy the next morning and found that all of the medicines were ready. This time, the labels had even been printed in English—they had never done that before. The people at the pharmacy called a taxi for us, and we went back to our hotel to pack the medicines into our suitcases.

Our last morning was spent in the usual way, at a little café across the street from our hotel. We sat at an outdoor table, sipping café crème and watching the Parisians hurrying to work. We knew we would miss Paris, but we also knew we'd be back in six months.

"Let me tell you the secret that has led me to my goal. My strength lies solely in my tenacity."

—LOUIS PASTEUR

CHAPTER NINE

Getting into Balance

We arrived home from Paris with renewed hope. It was always an emotional lift for me to be there and see Dr. Lapraz. I was able to start letting go of the fear, as he had suggested. I think that for the first time, I started having positive thoughts about my future. Obviously, none of us knows how much time we have left in this world, but I came back from Paris with the belief that Dr. Lapraz would be able to tell from my blood work when my body was getting into trouble. He would then be able to prescribe medicines that would help get me back into balance.

In Paris, Dr. Lapraz had suggested I find someone to work on the alignment of my body when I got back home. I decided to see Dr. Rook, my chiropractor. He's good with sports injuries, and had helped me a great deal in the past. At my first appointment with him it became obvious that the left side of my body was out of alignment because it hurt so much when he worked on that side. But it didn't hurt at all when he worked on my right side. He said that three appointments a week for three weeks were what I needed, and he was right.

Dr. Rook also gave me the name of a good yoga teacher, Cheri Clampett. She turned out to be one of the instructors at the Wellness Center, a program sponsored by the Cancer Center of Santa Barbara. They offered yoga classes three times a week—and they were free for cancer patients. What a deal! I found the classes amazing. I noticed a great feeling of positive energy when I entered the room. I think the fact that everyone in the class had cancer and was there to heal emotionally, as well as physically, gave us all an immediate bond.

The first hour of the class was dedicated to "Yoga for Strength and Empowerment." This class was ideal for women recovering from breast cancer, who had been weakened by cancer treatments. It became my favorite class. Flexibility postures, deep stretches, and standing poses were incorporated for total body conditioning and improving range of motion. The second hour of each class was called "Gentle Yoga for Health and Well-Being," which was much more gentle stretching and deep breathing to release tension in the body and quiet the mind.

Both classes are held three times a week with a different instructor. All of them are great and I try not to miss any of the sessions. I have learned a great deal from my teachers—Cheri, Kat and Anne—about how yoga can help me fight cancer. They've shown me which movements can support my immune system, which ones can help my liver, and which ones can stimulate and nourish different glands to restore balanced functioning.

But, most importantly, I gained an incredible support system by attending these yoga classes. I had never been interested in attending a discussion support group about cancer, although I know that it's important for some to have a place to go to talk about their fears and to be comforted. Yoga has become my support group. We naturally talk about how each person is doing before and after class. We call and email each other to find out how a medical test may have turned out. In the yoga classes I attend, we're all very positive and want to move forward. We're working to get our bodies back into shape and, to feel better physically and emotionally. It has become important to me to show those who are newly diagnosed, that they too can live with advanced cancer. I'm living proof.

Some people in yoga class are going through chemotherapy and they wear scarves, or wigs or are just bald. We've all been there. We're also there to cheer a person up after chemo, when little patches of hair start coming in, but not nearly as fast as hoped for. It was my yoga buddies who worried for me when my mother-in-law and father-in-law were hospitalized. They reminded me to take care of myself and asked about my in-laws at each class. We all have a bond and try to be there for each other when needed—like showing up when someone is going through chemotherapy to bring them a sandwich or a much-appreciated Popsicle. My yoga classes have been a real gift. I am so thankful that the Cancer Center of Santa Barbara understands what an important part these classes play in our recovery.

Since I no longer felt in "survival mode" I started to think about doing something about my breasts being two different sizes. My left breast had been made noticeably smaller years earlier by the surgery in which the tumor and surrounding tissue had been removed. I thought it might be nice to have the right breast made the same size as the left one. I thought it was a positive sign that I was even considering it.

My first step was to find out what Dr. Woliver thought about it, and ask for a referral for a plastic surgeon. He gave me the names of three surgeons he thought would be good for me to speak with. Next, I asked the people at the Wellness Center, where I took yoga, if they could give me a name. They referred me to the Breast Resource Center (BRC), which was located just a few blocks away. In general, the people I spoke with were excited that I was thinking about having the surgery.

I went to the BRC and spoke with the executive director. I had been meaning to visit the facility ever since reading an article about it in the local paper. The Center was set up in a little house near the hospital that had been converted into a comfortable place for cancer patients. The director was great and she told me all about the BRC. It seemed like a wonderful place for cancer patients to go to for advice, and to speak with other breast cancer survivors.

The BRC has many books for people to check out, and they conduct classes in disciplines such as Reiki, an ancient healing art. This gentle form of energy work promotes deep relaxation and has been found to reduce pain, relieve stress and promote recovery. A friend of mine with cancer has been very involved with Reiki and has found it to be extremely helpful. I left with lots of information about the Center. In addition, the director gave me the names of a few more plastic surgeons to put on my list.

I also called my gynecologist to see if she could refer me to a plastic surgeon. She suggested one in Los Angeles, but I didn't want to go out of town for what I thought would be a simple outpatient surgery. I called three of the names on my list and made appointments to see each of them.

Only one of the plastic surgeons I met with said that he would need to speak with Dr. Woliver to see if it was okay for me to go through the surgery. I liked this doctor very much and scheduled a second meeting where pre-surgery photographs would be taken to submit to my insurance company. I had already decided not to renew the lease on the small office I had rented after the sale of my company since most of the work regarding the sale had been completed. I was now working full time on my book, and thought that I would recover from the breast reconstruction surgery and work on the book at home and, therefore, wanted to schedule the surgery for some time after that. The next step was to wait and see if my insurance company would cover the cost of the surgery.

Around this time I decided to learn more about the doctor from New York who specialized in liver cancer that my girlfriend had told me about. I was curious to see if what he was doing would apply to my cancer. I had been told that he would need to see a recent CT scan and review my medical records before scheduling a consultation. But, before doing this I wanted to discuss it with Dr. Woliver.

Michael and I made an appointment with Dr. Woliver to go over the information we had compiled about this specialist, and to see what he thought. It was a very interesting meeting. Dr. Woliver told me that everything I showed him about this doctor and what he was doing for tumors of the liver was already being done at UCLA and the Cancer Center of Santa Barbara. He explained that the Cancer Center networked closely with UCLA. I hadn't known that before. He also told me that some of the procedures being discussed, such as cryosurgery and chemoembolization, wouldn't apply to my cancer since the tumors were scattered throughout my liver. He said that in those procedures, my entire liver would have to be treated, and that the treatments would be much more toxic than anything I had undergone thus far.

He said he didn't think it would hurt to go ahead and send a copy of my upcoming CT scan to this doctor in New York. Maybe they were doing something new that he wasn't aware of. Dr. Woliver mentioned that Xeloda was presently keeping me stable, but if it were to stop working, other things would have to be considered. None of us knew how long I would remain on Xeloda. At that time, I had been taking it longer than any of his other patients.

After meeting with Dr. Woliver, I realized that a special trip to New York really wasn't warranted at that time. I would send that doctor a copy of my upcoming CT scan and possibly schedule a meeting sometime when we were in the area. It was good to know what options existed if my cancer took a turn for the worse. I'm sure that I was hoping to learn that they were doing something entirely new and different—but they weren't. I went home feeling deflated. I was tired of blood work and taking all the pills I had to take. I guess I was just disappointed that this doctor wasn't doing anything really new.

I walked out on our deck and just allowed myself to feel those feelings. Michael saw me out at the railing and came over to put his arms around me. He could sense my emotions. We talked about how I was doing so well on Xeloda and the plant-based medicines. Why would I even want to consider doing anything else right now? I hadn't really thought it all through. When I did, I realized that trying something new might mean I would have had to go off Xeloda and the medicines from France, and I felt that would have been a huge mistake. I was stable and I wouldn't want to jeopardize that.

I also realized that I had been looking at other therapies out of concern about what would happen when Xeloda stopped working. I knew it was important to have a backup plan. Dr. Lapraz felt Xeloda was good in conjunction with the plant-based medicines he prescribed, and so I was worried about having to go on a different chemotherapy drug that wouldn't be as compatible with the medicines I was getting in France. Again, I had to let go of the fear of the unknown. It's so great that Michael and I can talk about these things openly. I just wish I could tape record Dr. Lapraz telling me to let go of the fear, and then listen to it every day!

The next morning I had my CT scan, and I asked them to fax me a copy of the written report. When I received the report, it showed that everything was still very stable—no new tumors. The report stated "Multiple hepatic lesions. Complex disease which is felt to be stable, particularly when compared with the study of 7/15/02"—about a year prior to this scan. My blood work also showed that I was in the normal range pretty much across the board (including tumor markers), except that my potassium level was down. Dr. Woliver wanted me to increase my intake of potassium supplements, and then have another blood test the following week.

Having a CT scan can bring up emotions about the realities of having cancer. At that time, I had a great deal on my mind. Thoughts kept swirling through my head about when Xeloda would stop working, whether or not I had started the plant-based medicines in time, and if having breast surgery was a good idea.

But, physically I had been feeling great, so, when I got a call from Cheryl suggesting that Michael and I take a little trip with them, I was elated. The timing couldn't have been better! Cheryl and Len had won a free trip for four people to a golf resort in Carmel, California in a raffle and wanted us to join them. How could we pass that up?

It was right around the time of Cheryl's and my birthday, so we decided to go to the resort for two days, and then drive to San Francisco, see Kim, and have a birthday weekend in the city of our birth. We had so much fun. A very funny thing happened in San Francisco. Kim wanted to surprise us, and baked a birthday cake to bring to the restaurant where we were having dinner with several other people. On the way there, the person giving her a ride made a sharp turn, and her hand ended up embedded in the cake. She was frantic when she arrived at the restaurant, and asked the Maitre d' to see if the chef could do something to make it presentable. The people at the restaurant couldn't have been nicer. When they brought the cake out, Kim was amazed. She said they made it look better than when it had left her kitchen! I think what made her feel the best, was when the chef sent word out that if any of the cake was left, he would love to have a piece. We were only too happy to oblige. Times like these are nice to be able to reflect on, and I knew then that we were fortunate to be experiencing them. Getting away really helped to clear my head.

For some time, I had subscribed to a daily email report called the Food and Drug Law Institute (FDLI) Smart Brief. It contains a synopsis of articles related to medical research that have appeared in various newspapers around the world.

In August 2003, the FDLI Smart Brief had a synopsis of an article from the Washington Post by Rob Stein reviewing the findings of a major study that found women who took any combination of estrogen and progestin were at risk for breast cancer. As I mentioned, I thought this combination had contributed to my cancer. Now it was being confirmed in the largest study ever done on hormone therapy—the Million Women Study. The findings were published in the British medical journal, The Lancet. The study involved more than one million British women aged 50-64 and followed them from 1996-2001. The results showed that women who took hormone replacement therapy (HRT), including estrogen-only and a combination of estrogen and progestin, faced an increased risk of breast cancer when compared with non-HRT users. Researchers found that postmenopausal women using combination HRT were twice as likely to develop breast cancer as women not on HRT, and that those only taking estrogen HRT increased their risk by 30 percent. However, the study showed that after stopping hormone therapy, the risk decreased, and after five years it reached the same level as the risk for women who didn't use HRT drugs.

The year before the Million Women Study came out, a landmark United States study by the Women's Health Initiative was stopped before it was completed because it was found that there was a significant risk of breast cancer for women who took HRT. One surprise finding was that the combination of estrogen and progestin failed to protect the heart and actually appeared to increase the risk for heart attacks, strokes and life-threatening blood clots. After these studies came out, public health authorities started to issue strong warnings regarding the use of HRT. The U.S. Food and Drug Administration strengthened warning labels on all hormone replacement therapy products, warning of the risk of heart disease, stroke and cancer. Some people say that one advantage of HRT is that it prevents bone fractures caused by osteoporosis. But the increased risk of heart disease and other health problems outweighs those benefits, according to FDA commissioner Dr. Mark McClellan. He also said that there are other drugs on the market that can prevent osteoporosis without the dangerous side effects of HRT. Recently, the U.S. government told makers of HRT products to add yet another warning to their labels, saying that HRT may increase older women's risk of Alzheimer's and other types of dementia.

Many women ignore the warnings about the risks of HRT because the hormones relieve hot flashes, mood swings, and other menopausal symptoms. I don't know the answer for everyone, but I would try acupuncture if I had hot flashes. I know women who have had great success with it. Most importantly, every woman should have a blood test to see what her levels of estrogen and progesterone are before considering any hormone therapy—either natural or synthetic. For example, if a woman has an overabundance of estrogen in her body, taking soy as a substitute for HRT could be very dangerous. She would be adding more estrogen to her body. That imbalance could put her at risk for breast cancer.

Shortly after returning from our trip to San Francisco, I received a call from the plastic surgeon's office saying that they had heard from my insurance company regarding the breast surgery. The insurance company had approved the surgery, and it was scheduled for September 11, 2003. I didn't think about the date until after I got off the phone. Then it hit me— 9/11 was a strange date to have surgery!

I suddenly realized that I hadn't emailed Dr. Lapraz about the breast surgery I was planning on having, so I wrote him all about it. He emailed me immediately expressing concern. He wanted to know what anesthesia would be used, and how long the surgery would last. He said he would need to start me on additional medicines as soon as I awoke from the anesthesia. I called the surgeon's office and spoke with the surgical nurse. I got the name of the anesthesia that would be used and found that the surgery would take from four and a half to five hours. I had an appointment set for the following week to go over all of this, but the nurse was very helpful and answered all of my questions.

Dr. Lapraz was even more concerned when he heard how long the surgery would last. He said it would be a major assault on my whole body. He was also afraid that my liver would become super reactive because of the anesthesia and post-operative shock. I explained that I really wanted this surgery, but that I would reconsider having it if he felt it would put me in danger. He told me he was against the surgery because he felt it could make the cancer in my liver unstable, and because it was not vital for me to have it. But he said that, since it was important to me, he would ask his colleague, Dr. Duraffourd, for a second opinion. Recently I learned that Dr. Duraffourd feels that anesthesia sharply modifies the reactivity of the hormonal system, and can cause a disease like cancer to spread.

I went to yoga the next day and told my friends that Dr. Lapraz was very much against my having the surgery. Chris, one of my friends in the class, called me at home later that night to discuss it. She said she had been worried about my having the surgery as well, since cancer was still present in my liver. She had spoken with her father, who was a retired surgeon, and he also had expressed concern.

I thought about what everyone was saying, and reread the emails from Dr. Lapraz. Then I discussed it all with Michael. I told him I had made a decision not to have the surgery, that it just wasn't worth the risk. He agreed completely. I then called Cheryl and told her. She was happy with my decision. I guess that many people had been concerned, but when they saw how excited I was about the idea of the surgery, they didn't say anything. I emailed Dr. Lapraz about my decision. He wrote me right back saying that Dr. Duraffourd had agreed with him regarding the danger of the surgery. They both were pleased I had decided against it. As they put it, "We are happy with your decision. It is a good one. Bravo!"

I since learned from Dr. Lapraz that general anesthesia could weaken the response of the immune system in terms of intensity and duration— functions of the endobiogenic state of the patient. Moreover, research has demonstrated that, among cancer patients, the removal of the main tumor can trigger the creation and diffusion of metastases within several weeks. This risk can be worsened by the temporary inhibiting impact of anesthesia on the immune system. That's why both Drs. Duraffourd and

Lapraz didn't want me to go through breast surgery. Although my stage four cancer was stabilized, they felt the risk was too high, when the surgery wasn't necessary for my health. They had seen too many stabilized cancers spread in a matter of months (and sometimes weeks) after patients had undergone surgery.

I called the plastic surgeon's office and told the receptionist that I needed to speak with him about the concerns that had been raised by my doctor in Paris regarding the surgery. He called me right back, and as soon as he heard about how Dr. Lapraz felt, he also said that we shouldn't do the surgery. He agreed with Dr. Lapraz that the surgery could throw my body out of balance, so why take the risk. He was wonderful, and told me that if I ever just needed to talk with someone, that he would always be available. He said he admired how I had handled my cancer, and that it was an honor to have met me. I surely didn't expect to hear that from a doctor I had only seen twice. He was obviously one of the special ones!

After all of the dust settled, I reflected on the whole situation. It had really been very unlike me to have considered undergoing surgery that wasn't totally necessary. The thought that I might have put my life in danger was scary. I had worked hard to be in balance, had finally lost 20 pounds, and was feeling great. Having two breasts the same size just wasn't important enough to risk it all. It's not like it's obvious to anyone but me. I know many women who have had mastectomies and then went on to have breast reconstruction. That's a different thing. Usually those women don't have fourth-stage breast cancer. Their doctors probably thought that the cancer had been removed with the tumor and surrounding tissue. My cancer was still there, and at the moment, wasn't active. Why should I risk stirring it up?

Then in October 2003 it was time for our next trip to Paris. This time it would again be a "twin trip"—meaning that our husbands were going to sit it out. I was anxious to see what my blood test results would be since a whole year had passed since I sold my company. I remembered that at our last appointment, Dr. Lapraz said more time was needed without stress before changes would show up in the Biology of Functions. I also couldn't wait to step on the scales and show Dr. Lapraz how much weight I had lost since our last trip.

The clinical exam at Dr. Lapraz's office couldn't have been better. Not only had Cheryl and I each lost more than ten pounds since our last visit (which also meant decreasing the levels of estrogen in my body), but I was also more in balance. During my last visit, the left side of my body had been blocked because of my broken toe. Now, as a result of the medicines, yoga and acupressure, my body was in better shape than it had ever been before.

While we were at his office, Dr. Lapraz phoned his friend, Patrice Pauly, who had been working with him on a book about endobiogénie. He asked Patrice if he could come by the office to meet me. When Patrice arrived, we spoke about the book I was writing and how he might help me with technical details regarding endobiogénie. Cheryl and I made a follow-up appointment with Dr. Lapraz for a few days later, when the blood tests would be back from the lab. We left his office elated.

That trip to Paris turned out to be full of great news. When the lab results came back, they showed that my tumor markers were down and that everything was much improved. Dr. Lapraz said there was virtually no inflammation in my body. When I stepped out of his office to use the restroom, Dr. Lapraz said to Cheryl, "Carol is going to live!" For the first time, it seemed he felt that I wasn't in imminent danger.

But the following year, many things changed. I experienced great stress after the deaths of several important people in my life: my father-in-law, Lou; a very close friend from yoga, Chris Dahl; and the person who had purchased my company, Dale Byars. To top it all off, we lost our beloved

Rottweiler, Riley, to cancer. That stress, coupled with the fact that I was not being attentive to my diet and bodily changes caused by the end of menopause once again activated the cancer in my liver. More on that distressing news in just a bit.

But, not all the news was bad that year. I had been concerned that once my book was published many people who wanted to consult Dr. Lapraz would find it difficult to travel to Paris. That's why I was glad to hear that he was now training doctors in the United States in endobiogénie, and they expected to open a clinic in the state of Idaho in the near future. That clinic did open in Pocatello, Idaho in December 2004.

The person most responsible for bringing Dr. Lapraz to the United States is a wonderful woman named Annemarie Buhler. She is one of the founders of Time Laboratories, a company that has produced therapeutic-quality natural products since 1972. Working to forward the research and understanding of phyto-aromatherapy, Ms. Buhler established the Phyto-Aromatherapy Institute (PAI) in 1992 with Drs. Duraffourd and Lapraz. Since then the Institute has since hosted numerous Endobiogenic Concept™ medical seminars in the United States. Led by Dr. Lapraz, these seminars have been aimed at educating American physicians and other health professionals in the use of medicinal plants.

It was at one of these seminars in Pocatello, Idaho in September 2004 that I met Dr. Jean Bokelmann. I had been asked to speak about my experiences with cancer and the ways in which endobiogénie had helped to stabilize my disease. Dr. Bokelmann was one of the attendees at that seminar. She sat right across from me and I could see that she was completely engrossed in everything Dr. Lapraz was saying. When I was introduced to her later, I found her to be so very open and warm. She told me that my story had brought tears to her eyes, as a friend of hers was battling breast cancer. I knew then and there that a great team was in the making—she and Dr. Lapraz were meant to work together!

Dr. Bokelmann is a graduate of Stanford University and Case Western Reserve University School of Medicine. An Associate Professor of Family Medicine and Geriatrics at Idaho State University, she has been on the faculty of Idaho State University's Family Practice Residency Program since its inception in 1992. She has been director of the Student Health Center at ISU since 1995. Dr. Bokelmann told me how impressed she was by the intricate scientific basis of endobiogénie, and that she felt compelled to learn more about it. She decided that she wanted to assist Dr. Lapraz in bringing this field of medicine to the United States.

Since 2004, Drs. Duraffourd and Lapraz have been training Dr. Bokelmann in endobiogénie, and they continue to consult with her on individual cases. She now sees patients at the Endobiogenic Integrative Medical Center (EIMC) in Pocatello. The EIMC is a collaborative endeavor between Idaho State University, Annemarie Buhler, and Drs. Lapraz and Duraffourd. The creation of the Center was a huge step forward in bringing this valuable diagnostic and therapeutic tool to more patients. Today, Dr. Lapraz travels to Idaho every three to six months in order to train doctors in endobiogénie, and to work with Dr. Bokelmann at the EIMC where he also sees his American patients.

Now back to the story of the reactivated cancer in my liver. A routine CT scan in December 2004 showed that there were two new lesions in my liver, although the rest of the tumors were unchanged. Dr. Woliver put me back on a schedule of two weeks on Xeloda and only one week off (I had been on a schedule of two weeks on and two weeks off for the previous three years), and Drs. Lapraz and Duraffourd changed my plant-based medicines. Another CT scan done in March 2005 showed that the tumors in my liver were again stable and, thankfully, that there were no new lesions. It appeared the changes we made were working.

By my tenth visit to Paris in May 2005, my disease appeared to be on the road to stability after a very stressful year. I had been working hard to reduce the stress in my life, but I didn't feel I was yet in the clear since my tumor markers were still elevated. The good news was that I felt great! I learned a valuable lesson and that was if you do get out of balance, it's possible to get back into balance. I tucked that away for future reference!

"Courage is like love—it must have hope to nourish it."

—NAPOLÉON BONAPARTE

CHAPTER TEN

Losing My Hair—Again!

In June 2005 a CT scan showed that three of the tumors in my liver had increased in size. There were no new lesions, but the report now called it "progressive liver mets." The rest of my body seemed to be in balance and I felt fine, but the tumors were obviously becoming a concern. In spite of the new activity in the liver, Dr. Woliver and I decided that I would stay on a schedule of two weeks on Xeloda and one week off. Through correspondence with Drs. Lapraz and Duraffourd I learned that my body was still going through hormonal changes due to menopause, and that my estrogen levels still needed to come down.

A big love of mine is golf, and I decided it would be good to get back into playing regularly in order to get more balance in my life. My time had been so tied up with the cancer center and writing my book, that I needed something to take me to a completely different place mentally. Golf did that for me. When I'm on a golf course, surrounded by rolling green grass and listening to birds sing, I don't think about anything but hitting that little white ball (with a pink ribbon imprinted on it, of course)!

My son, Michael, had proposed to his girlfriend, Lisa, and the wedding was set for December 31, 2005 in Bend, Oregon. It was going to be a very exciting New Year's Eve. Lisa is a wonderful girl, and she's such a perfect match for my son. I couldn't wait for her to join our family. Michael and I decided to visit Michael and Lisa in Bend during August, and we went wedding gown shopping—that was so much fun!

While we were in Bend, Michael and I both fell in love with the wonderful town and the beauty of the surrounding area. A great ski resort at Mt. Bachelor is just minutes away from the city, and pine trees are everywhere you look! The Deschutes River runs through the middle of a beautiful downtown, which is full of great restaurants and shops. I remember Michael turning to me and saying that we should think about buying a house here where we could retire one day! The idea stuck, and three weeks later we flew back to Bend to look at houses. We found a wonderful home on three pine-filled acres just outside of town. Unfortunately, we had to cut the trip short when we heard that Michael's mother, Esther, had passed away. It was a blessing for her—she had deteriorated considerably since her stroke, didn't know who anyone was, and couldn't speak or eat. We both knew that she was now with dad—they were inseparable in life and we believe they are together again now.

So, that August was a mixed bag. We discovered the beauty of Bend, Oregon, but there was also the sad passing of my mother-in-law, who I loved so very much. Another high point that month came when my book was finally completed and went to press. It was so amazing to see the first copy—I couldn't wait for it to be in bookstores!

Dr. Lapraz was scheduled to conduct a seminar in Pocatello in October. Annette Davis (Annemarie Buhler's granddaughter who runs the EIMC) asked if I would speak at the seminar, and then follow with a book signing. I also agreed to speak at a public lecture in Pocatello and do another book signing there. After the seminar, a television news anchor for a local station asked if Drs. Lapraz and Bokelmann and I would be available for an interview on a program called "Ask the Doc" hosted by Dr. Curtis Galke.

I happily agreed. It was fun and there were lots of calls from viewers asking about endobiogénie.

It's important to point out that Annette Davis, who is a certified nutritionist, works closely with Dr. Bokelmann at the EIMC as they see and evaluate patients. I have been truly amazed by the knowledge about plants and their medicinal value that Annette has acquired through her training, and her family's long association with Dr. Lapraz. For example, on several occasions I've asked Annette about an article I've read touting the benefits of some herb or dietary supplement for cancer patients. She describes the particular action of the herb or supplement in question, and then explains why it might or might not be beneficial for someone in my situation. She always reminds me that what is good for one person may not be good for another, and that without special knowledge and training it is very difficult to know the difference.

During this time, three of the tumors in my liver had been growing. I accepted Dr. Lapraz's explanation that this was because of hormonal changes that were taking place in my body. Nevertheless, it was something that had to be dealt with. Dr. Woliver said that we might need to think about changing my chemotherapy. I had been on Xeloda for almost five years, and he pointed out that it might have done as much as it was going to do for me. Still, I really didn't want to try something new before my son's wedding. With that big event coming up, I didn't want to have to worry about low white counts or feeling sick. So, it was decided that I would I stay on Xeloda until after the wedding. A November CT scan showed the liver lesions were stable with no new ones in evidence. That meant that I was able to turn to thoughts of the upcoming wedding.

We had Thanksgiving at our new home in Bend that year. It was wonderful to look out at all the trees and watch the deer run up and down the hill outside our window. Our son, David, came for Thanksgiving, as did Cheryl and Len. They all fell in love with the beauty of Central Oregon!

Then before we knew it, it was December and time to drive back to Bend for the wedding! We went skiing at Mt. Bachelor on Christmas Day. The mountain was empty because the weather was so cold and windy. It was a whiteout at the top and I got what felt like a strong dose of altitude sickness! I hadn't skied since I had been on chemotherapy, so I really couldn't be sure what made me feel so light-headed. While feeling light-headed, I fell and got a cut across the top of my nose where my goggles hit my face. Besides the cut, I ended up with two black eyes—just six days before the wedding! Fortunately, several days later and with a little make-up, all was fine. As I've mentioned before, we all need to laugh to stimulate our immune system. At the time, however, it didn't seem very funny. But now that I look back, it seems like an episode from a 1950's sitcom! A few days before my son's wedding, Michael and I celebrated our 10th wedding anniversary.

The wedding was so beautiful. There was snow all along the River running behind the hotel where the ceremony and reception took place. I thought about when I had first been diagnosed with cancer and only given a couple of years to live. It seemed that I would not be there to see my son get married, but yet here I was! I've never been one to dwell on the negative. I just thought that it was possible, and it was! Michael and Lisa surprised us by having the song that we danced to at our wedding played, and invited us out on the dance floor. What a truly magical day it turned out to be!

After we returned to Santa Barbara in January 2006, a CT scan showed that three of the lesions in my liver had grown, but there were no new ones and my spleen was unchanged. Dr. Woliver talked to Michael and me about going off of Xeloda and onto a drug called Doxil. This was shortly before Dr. Lapraz was scheduled to come to Santa Barbara from

Paris to meet Dr. Woliver and go over my latest blood work and CT scan. So, we decided to wait until we could all meet before making a decision about Doxil. Dr. Jean Bokelmann also came from Pocatello for the meeting. I had arranged for the use of a conference room at a local hotel and had invited several other local doctors to meet Dr. Lapraz and hear about endobiogénie. This informal conference took place after our meeting with Dr. Woliver. At that meeting everyone agreed that I should go off of Xeloda and start Doxil the following week. After the meeting, a local television news anchor named Debby Davison interviewed the doctors for a special feature that her station would air later in the month. She came to my house the following week to interview me and get film of me taking my endobiogenic medicines and tea. Debby did an incredible job putting the piece together, and I got calls from so many people who saw it and were impressed. The common comment was that "it was like something you'd see on national TV, not a local station!" Debby has since semi-retired, and we've stayed in touch and I value her friendship.

The day after Drs. Lapraz and Bokelmann spoke in Santa Barbara, Michael and I drove them to Los Angeles, where they met with Dr. Stephen Vasilev, a prominent oncologist. Drs. Lapraz and Vasilev had a patient in common, and had met once before. Dr. Lapraz also met with Dr. Bill Tap, an oncologist at UCLA, and a few other oncologists. It was a busy weekend for him and Dr. Bokelmann. I heard afterwards that most of the doctors were very interested and would like to do research with Dr. Lapraz.

As we had planned, I went off of Xeloda and started Doxil on January 23, 2006. Doxil is a version of Adriamycin, which is a strong chemotherapy drug I had been given when first diagnosed with metastatic breast cancer in November 1999. However, Doxil is eliminated more slowly than Adriamycin, because the active agent is encased in tiny fat molecules that are carried throughout the body before being metabolized. The hope was that this would allow Doxil to have the same strong effect as Adriamycin, while causing fewer side effects. A study of 509 women, half of whom were treated with Doxil and half with Adriamycin, showed that significantly fewer women taking Doxil had heart problems, hair loss, vomiting, or reduced white blood cell counts. Yet it was deemed just as effective for treating metastatic breast cancer. Well, that sure sounded great to me! I was scheduled to have it every four weeks and then would have a CT scan at the end of two months.

While I was happy that I wouldn't have to worry about hair loss and low white counts, going on the new drug was an adjustment. I would now be going into the cancer center every four weeks for an infusion, rather than just taking medication in pill form as I had been doing for the past five years. But, it did appear that the cancer was active again, and we needed to see if we could stabilize it! This was an emotional change for me, but we had been talking about it for many months so it wasn't really a surprise. Emotionally, I felt that I was taking a step backwards by having to go into the chemo room for the infusions. I had often visited other patients who were friends of mine when they were having chemo. I would talk to the chemo nurses and they would tell me how great it was to see me doing so well. Now I was going to be one of their patients again. But it was simply what I had to do, so I made the adjustment!

Around this time, our friends from Paris, Danny and Patrice Pauly and their daughter Gwénaëlle, came to visit us in Santa Barbara. Gwénaëlle was in her mid-twenties and had arranged to do a five-month internship at Michael's graphic design firm. She would be living with us during the internship. Aside from getting professional experience as a graphic designer, she wanted to learn to speak English more fluently. I was looking forward to her stay. After the five of us enjoyed a few days in Santa Barbara, Danny and Patrice flew to Hawaii for a two-week vacation. After Hawaii, they met us at our home in Bend before returning to France.

After my second infusion of Doxil, we took the now-familiar drive to Oregon with Gwénaëlle and the dogs. As expected, I didn't have any real side effects from the chemotherapy, which was a huge relief! I didn't lose my hair and my white count stayed high. We had a wonderful time showing our friends around Bend and the surrounding areas. They particularly loved a quaint little town called Sisters. It's located just a few miles from Bend and has the feel of someplace straight out of the old West.

The time went fast and we were soon saying goodbye to our friends and heading back to Santa Barbara. After two cycles on Doxil, I was scheduled to have a CT scan to see how it was working. Unfortunately, the results were not what we had hoped for. The report from the radiologist said that there had been progression of disease in the liver with the development of multiple new lesions! This was a real surprise to me. I had started on Doxil and stopped taking Xeloda because three existing tumors had grown while I was on Xeloda. But at least Xeloda had kept any new tumors from developing. Now, after just a short time on Doxil I had multiple new tumors!

We met with Dr. Woliver to discuss our next step. He thought I should go back on Xeloda in combination with the chemotherapy Gemzar (Gemcitabine) I knew others who had good results with Gemzar. I also knew that it was considered a gentle chemo that works by interfering with the process by which cells divide and repair themselves. This action would hopefully prevent the further growth of cancer cells and lead to their death. Dr. Woliver said that his other patients on Gemzar usually didn't lose their hair, but that it could cause thinning of the hair and a low white count. The schedule for Gemzar was infusions for two weeks in a row and then one week off.

I started back on Xeloda that same day and my first infusion of Gemzar was four days later. The next week, during my second infusion, the chemo really started to cause pain in my veins. They chemo nurses helped me manage it by keeping a warm blanket over my arm during the infusion.

I had been told that, because of this problem, it would be best to have a port (port-a-cath) installed when receiving infusions of Gemzar. A port is a device that allows easy access to the main blood supply for patients who frequently receive intravenous infusions. It consists of a small reservoir compartment and a plastic tube, or catheter, which is surgically inserted into a vein. The whole device is placed under the skin of the upper chest between the collarbone and the breast, where it appears as a little bump about the size of a quarter. The surgery to install a port is considered minor, and is done with just a local anesthetic. During chemotherapy, the nurse inserts a needle into the port instead of having to find a vein. This can be a good solution for people who have ongoing problems with the nurse finding a good vein. Blood tests can also be taken from the port, making that process easier. But at this point I wasn't sure if Gemzar was going to work for me, so I didn't see the sense in having a port put in. For all I knew, the next thing we would try could be a hormone therapy that wouldn't be given intravenously.

The blood test I had just before my third infusion of Gemzar showed that my white count was too low for chemo. I had to have Neupogen shots for two days in a row in order to bring the counts up before I could have that next infusion of Gemzar. Thankfully, there was a new procedure at the cancer center and now there was just one person giving the shots. She made sure the vials of Neupogen were warmed up before giving the injection, and that made it totally painless. I also had gotten some mouth sores while on Gemzar, but I felt fine otherwise and my energy level was not affected at all. I credit that to the plant-based medicines I had been taking from Dr. Lapraz.

At the end of April, I had another CT scan to see how the Gemzar and Xeloda were working. Unfortunately, they weren't working at all! The report said there was further progression of the disease, that numerous masses had increased in size, and that there were new lesions in both lobes of the liver. WOW—that was the worse CT scan report I had received thus far! I really started to think that the chemotherapy was doing exactly the opposite what it was supposed to be doing. It seemed to me that it was activating the cancer instead of stopping its progression.

I sent an email to my friend Colleen to let her know that the Gemzar wasn't working. Her response was an amazing comfort at the time, and the knowledge she imparted stayed with me as I continued on my search for the right combination of drugs to keep the cancer at bay. I'm including her email below (with her permission) because I want those with cancer to know that supporting one another can be so powerful, and can give hope and comfort during a very stressful time:

Dear Carol,

I've had some friends do very well with Avastin.... A girlfriend of mine was on an Avastin trial where her 3 cm breast cancer was first given Avastin, then AC (Adriamycin/Cytoxan) followed by Taxol prior to surgery. It was gone! Neither oncologist nor surgeon can find it to the point they don't have to do a mastectomy, just a simple lumpectomy. I also have a girlfriend whose tumor markers have been climbing for 3 years getting around 3200. She was put on Abraxane and it dropped down to 2300...first time in 3 years and almost a 1000 pts. ...

I know you don't want to be go through "hard core" chemo...but side effects nowadays have more options to dismiss them, both homeopathically, integrative and with new medications than they did 6-7 yrs ago. I read last night "God rather put us in situations where by his help we can develop virtues.... that the best answers to prayers may be the vision and strength to meet a circumstance or to assume a responsibility," By C.R. Findley. Aren't you looking for ways that integrated services (acupuncture to homeopathic) to relieve and ease a patient going through chemo? You want to write about it.... in my opinion; your book was so widely received because you "experienced" first hand homeopathic oncology. You believe in it...and I believe a marriage of both Western & European medicine will "both" keep us alive to develop old age!

It's hard facing fear that the cancer is growing after all these years. Try to remember that within every crisis there is an opportunity. I truly believe you're back in that tunnel, but you'll find another way out and let others know how to find the sunshine again.

Love you and let me know if I can help in any way,

Colleen

After the CT scan, Michael and I met with Dr. Woliver to discuss our next plan of attack. He thought I should go off Gemzar but stay on Xeloda and try a hormone therapy called Faslodex. Faslodex is given as an intramuscular injection once a month. When I asked Dr. Lapraz's opinion via email, he said that since I still had a lot of estrogen in my body that was feeding the tumors that Faslodex sounded like a good option. I learned that Faslodex is an anti-estrogen agent that produces anti-cancer effects through two mechanisms. First, it binds to estrogen receptors on individual cells, crowding out the estrogen. Second, Faslodex degrades the estrogen receptors to which it is bound. Both of these mechanisms prevent cancer cells from accessing enough estrogen for cellular growth and replication. Research has shown that people who haven't responded to Tamoxifen or another aromatase inhibitor could still respond to Faslodex.

The day after the meeting with Dr. Woliver, I flew to Pocatello for an appointment with Dr. Lapraz. I could see he was very concerned about what the chemotherapy was doing to my body. He changed my endobiogenic medicines and repeated that he agreed with Dr. Woliver that it was best to go off Gemzar and try Faslodex in conjunction with Xeloda.

I was concerned because I am deathly afraid of intramuscular injections! But I just concentrated on the fact that it couldn't possibly hurt as much as I was anticipating it would. I knew I would get through it, but it still wore on my mind. When I went in for the injection the nurse said, "Do you want me to freeze the area first, or should we just go for it?" I said why not use the freeze. The freeze is Ethyl Chloride, which is a topical anesthetic skin refrigerant, and it totally numbed the area. I didn't feel the shot at all! I couldn't believe it. I learned later that if the injection is given in the upper part of the buttocks you can sit afterwards without feeling a thing! That first shot didn't hurt when I got it, but the nurse gave it to me right in the middle of the butt so it was painful to sit down for the rest of that day. Talk about stress reduction for the shots that would follow! I ended up getting a booster injection two weeks later so we could jump-start the effect of the Faslodex. I would have freaked out if I hadn't known that the injections would be painless!

It was hard to believe, but Gwénaëlle had now been with us for five months and her internship at Michael's office was over. She had decided to go back to Brussels, where she had attended a university. We all enjoyed her stay and I think she learned a lot—and her English was much improved!

In all, I got four Faslodex injections. Then it was time for a CT scan, which was scheduled for July 18, 2006—one day before my 60th birthday. This was not a good birthday present! The report said there were multiple new lesions and the existing tumors had grown considerably. The report also noted that the liver remained enlarged and there was an enlarging lesion at the tip of the liver. One strange thing was that the report said the lobulated low-density lesion in my spleen had decreased considerably in size. We had always considered that to be a non-cancerous lesion and now we had to re-think that conclusion! I have to say that I believe the medicines from France kept me feeling just fine with no pain.

No one would ever guess that I had such advanced metastatic breast cancer if they looked at me! I think the rest of my organs were in balance.

There was one bright spot that day when I logged on to amazon.com and saw a new review for my book that had been written by a total stranger. It was so uplifting and it made me feel so great to know that my book continued to help others. What a nice time to see that review!

Again, it was time for a discussion with Dr. Woliver, and we weren't sure which direction to take. In addition to the CT scan, we talked about my most recent blood tests, which showed that one of my primary tumor markers (CA15-3) continued to go up. It was now 552 (the normal range is below 30).

At a previous meeting, Dr. Woliver had mentioned that one potential therapy would be a combination of two different drugs—a low-dose oral methotrexate (MTX) and cyclophosphamide, which is known as Cytoxan (CTX). The methotrexate would be taken daily and Cytoxan two times a week. Cytoxan has been around for quite some time. It is an anti-cancer drug that works by interfering with the growth of malignant cells. In combination with Cytoxan, the low-dose methotrexate was expected to work as an antiangiogensis agent. That is to say that it would inhibit the growth of new blood vessels, which cancerous tumors need to survive. Dr. Woliver told me that if I did go on MTX and CTX, I would need to go off of Xeloda. That was a no-brainer since my old friend Xeloda didn't seem to be doing anything for me anyway!

I got an email from Dr. Lapraz about my latest blood work. He said:

> "Your biology of functions shows clearly you have an excess of estro and folliculinic and androgenic activity which increases the development of cancer cells. So we need to immediately decrease these excessive activities.
>
> What I propose is to use Triptorelin which inhibits estrogen activity but not in the same way as Faslodex; it blocks central pituitary activity and

inhibits the development of receptors to estrogens, and that is a different mechanism then that of Faslodex, and in your case as you are also presenting an excess of prolactinic activity which in the same effect, all together with FSH excess increases the number of receptors to estrogens, these medicines seem to be more adapted for the moment. So we need to block all these hormonal excesses at the same time: at central and peripheral level, and also decrease androgenic activity.

I think, if Dr Woliver agrees, you could have the Triptorelin injections and an aromatase inhibitor (such as Aromasin) as well as taking the Cytoxan and Methotrexate."

I had been on an aromatase inhibitor (Femara) before, but that was a non-steroidal aromatase inhibitor, and Aromasin is a steroidal aromatase inhibitor. Research has shown people that do not have a good response to one can respond to the other. I emailed Dr. Woliver about what Dr. Lapraz proposed. Dr. Woliver responded that he was not that familiar with Triptorelin being used for postmenopausal women but would check into it. Dr. Lapraz had also asked me to mention to Dr. Woliver that he was worried about my FSH/LH being too active. FSH (Follicle Stimulating Hormone) is a hormone that stimulates an increase in estrogen secretion. LH (Luteinizing Hormone) is another hormone that also increases the production of progesterone and androgen. He wrote:

"Depending on my understanding of your case, I think it is necessary to block your FSH and LH and that Triptorelin was indicated because your FSH/LH activity is too active as we can see on your biology of functions, and this activity is increasing liver receptors to estrogens and androgens, in relationship with prolactine receptors, which are feeding your tumors. Can you ask Dr. Woliver if he is not worried about several effects of aromasin: stimulation of FSH and LH, and androgenic effects (even light). But as you know, your androgenic and estrogenic activity is yet too high."

Dr. Lapraz was worried that if I did start taking Aromasin but not Triptorelin, it would stimulate my FSH and LH. That could be a big mistake. Dr. Woliver agreed that Triptorelin made sense and said he would order the injection.

I mention this incident because it shows how much both Drs. Woliver and Lapraz were on top of my various treatments. During this time I'm sure it was very difficult for Dr. Lapraz to keep reevaluating my endobiogenic medicines because my chemotherapies and hormone therapies were changing so fast! Endobiogenic medicines need time to take effect in the body and are not normally changed so frequently. Dr. Lapraz kept reevaluating regularly his endobiogenic treatments in line with my Biology response to hormonal and chemotherapy treatments.

Eight days after the Triptorelin injection, a new set of blood tests showed that my CA15-3 shot up to 1020 (from 552 in the previous test). It also showed that the levels of a couple of liver enzymes that were usually in the normal range had become really high! The AST was 345 (normal is 0-41) and the ALT was 366 (normal is 5-45). I knew that Triptorelin could initially cause something called tumor flare, but both Drs. Woliver and Lapraz thought that the increase was linked to my breast cancer and not a side effect of the new therapies. Dr. Woliver wanted to get a CT scan done to see what was going on in the liver. I loved the email I got from him in response to my email talking about the high tumor markers. He said:

> "It is hard to remain positive yet there is no reason to panic. We might need to make some hard decisions about chemotherapy depending on the results of the scan."

I was so grateful to have such an incredible team of doctors working on my behalf. I also received an extremely positive email about the high tumor markers from Dr. Bokelmann at the EIMC. She wrote:

"You're right—we have a challenge ahead. You've faced this challenge before. The cancer has a different face than previously, so it's just a matter of trying to figure out its personality. What do you think Tom (Dr. Woliver) will suggest next? I recall that you mentioned a couple of options before. I'm sending positive thoughts your way. It's so easy to feel pessimistic at a time like this –and so important to stay positive and determined and powerful. You have so much inner power still. I'm feeling positive."

How lucky I am that she's part of my team! It wasn't until six months later that I came across the studies that Norman Cousins did at UCLA Medical School on how important the physician/patient relationship is in determining how well a patient responds to therapy. I wish every physician would read his book *"Head First: The Biology of Hope and the Healing Power of the Human Spirit."*

My body was trying to adjust to all the different drugs. One unfortunate side effect was an overnight weight gain of six pounds! This was so disturbing to me, yet I knew that losing weight was something my doctors would be more concerned about. Thankfully after a couple of days the excess weight left as quickly as it came. It was an emotional time and I'm sure my hormones were all over the place!

A September 7, 2006 CT scan showed there was further progression of multiple metastatic lesions in the liver. The lesion at the tip of the liver had grown considerably, and there was new evidence of a lesion extending from the liver to the head of the pancreas. Strangely enough, the lesion in the spleen had decreased in size again and was now less than 1 cm! I guess the tumor in the spleen responded to hormone therapy better than chemotherapy because it reduced in size when I got the Faslodex injections and now to the Aromasin and the Triptorelin. But the rest of the tumors clearly had not responded to any of the therapies we had tried over the past eight months.

I'm sure this is all very overwhelming to readers who have metastatic breast cancer. But it's important to know that there are many choices and it's just a matter of finding the right combination of therapies for each person. What works for one may not work for another—remember, we are all so very different. Please don't be disturbed to hear that Doxil, or Gemzar, or Faslodex didn't work for me when they have for many other cancer patients. Xeloda worked for me for nearly five years, and it has continued to work even longer for my friend Colleen. Yet other cancer patients I know have had no success with Xeloda. As I've learned from endobiogénie, our bodies are all so individual that we require different therapies to bring them back into balance and stabilize our disease. It's times like this that we just need to dig deep and find the confidence that we can do it.

I always go to the radiologist's office and pick up a copy of my CT scan report on the same day that I have the scan. As soon as I got this one, I emailed Dr. Woliver to say I could see that things didn't look good. I told him that I was mentally ready to start on weekly infusions of a stronger chemotherapy drug called Abraxane. This was something we had previously discussed. Abraxane is commonly used to treat breast cancer after failure of combination chemotherapy for metastatic disease. I also asked him if we should continue with the Triptorelin injections because of the FSH/LH. He wrote back saying that he strongly believed it was time to abort hormonal therapy, and that he felt we couldn't afford to wait the requisite time that would be needed to judge its effectiveness. He added if there was a response to Abraxane we could reconsider using hormonal therapy to maintain a remission off of chemo. Again, there was that positive thinking ahead about "maintaining a remission off of chemo!" This is exactly the sort of thing doctors need to do in order to help their patients stay mentally positive!

At my appointment with Dr. Woliver several days later, I was experiencing a great deal of pain in the area around my liver. It was even painful to the touch. After examining me, Dr. Woliver said my liver was enlarged and it wasn't unusual for someone in my situation to experience pain from sudden stretching of the capsule surrounding the liver. I had my first infusion of the Abraxane on September 13, 2006. My new weekly schedule would be to draw blood on Monday to be sure my blood counts (the CBC) were up so I could have the Abraxane Tuesday morning. Then on Wednesday, Thursday and Friday I would go to the cancer center for a Neupogen shot to keep my white counts up so I wouldn't be susceptible to infection. Low white counts are a common side effect of Abraxane. This schedule soon became very routine.

I emailed Dr. Lapraz about the pain I was having. I explained that a pain that felt like a muscle spasm had awakened me at 4:00 in the morning, and that it was hard for me to take a deep breath. He wrote back and told me that he believed that the pain was linked to a blockage of my liver's eliminatory function. He wanted me to drink an herbal tea made from *combretum raimbaultii* and *Melissa officinalis*. I found out later that he had chosen those two plants for their fluidizing effects on the secretion of liver bile, and in order to induce the sphincter that controls secretions from the liver to allow more fluid to pass.

I found the *Melissa officinalis* (which is also known as lemon balm) at a local health food store, but couldn't locate *combretum raimbaultii*. Since Dr. Lapraz was planning to come to Los Angeles within the week and would be seeing me there, he said he would try to bring some with him. In the meantime, I was to brew the *Melissa officinalis* tea and drink a cup of the tea every two hours. To brew it I put 4 tablespoons of the dry herb into a liter of water, brought it to a boil for 15 minutes, and then let it infuse for another 15 minutes. As I said, I drank a cup of it every two hours. I did just as he suggested and within a day I was totally amazed to be feeling like a whole new person!

But just as that discomfort cleared up, I got a new pain in my right shoulder. In an email Dr. Woliver said it was most likely what is called referred pain, and was being caused by the liver irritating the right side of my diaphragm. I was scheduled to see Dr. Lapraz in Los Angeles in just a couple of days and hoped that he would have some remedy for the pain in my upper back. After examining me, Dr. Lapraz did a very deep tissue massage on my back in order to alleviate some of the congestion that I had. He explained that this sort of deep tissue massage would result in relaxation of the muscles that had become tight and stiff because of congestion in my liver. After that massage, I was so sore that I couldn't bear to sit against anything for a couple of days, but the pain in my upper back was gone and I was feeling so much better.

My next chemo session was just a week after the last time I had just seen Dr. Woliver in his office. That was when it had been so painful to even have him touch the area around my liver. After that is when I did the Melissa tea and had my exam with Dr. Lapraz. At that next chemo session, Dr. Woliver came into the room to see how I was doing. I was happy to tell him that I felt great! He just couldn't believe the transformation that had transpired in just one week. I had emailed him about the tea, telling him how much better I felt afterwards, but it was seeing me looking so good and pain free that seemed to astonish him. He said he needed to understand more of what Dr. Lapraz is doing! Another amazing thing about Dr. Woliver is his openness to what Dr. Lapraz is doing for me. I guess seeing is believing!

By the end of September 2006, my CA15-3 was at an all-time high of 1440. But, my liver enzymes were coming down and I tried not to be too worried about it. I knew it would take at least two full sessions of Abraxane to get a good indication of how I was responding to it. I also remembered back to Colleen's email about a friend of hers whose tumor markers had gotten over 3000 before going on Abraxane. I think this is an important thing for cancer patients to remember—your markers can get high, but they can also come back down.

After the second infusion of Abraxane, my hair started to thin out. Since I wasn't sure if it would just stay thin or completely fall out, I got a fall. That really helped with the transition, because within a month I could tell I was going to be completely bald! This was an emotional time, but probably not as emotional as the first time I had lost my hair nearly seven years earlier. My twin sister, Cheryl, told me she had heard of cancer patients going to a wig maker in Los Angeles, who had made them wigs that fit perfectly. That had been a problem the first time I lost my hair. My head is rather small, and the ready-made wigs that were available didn't stay on very well and tended to irritate my scalp. I knew that this time around I also wanted to get a wig made out of human hair. Synthetic wigs can be damaged very easily by heat from a stove or oven, or a fireplace. I found that out the first time around, when I singed the synthetic wig I had at the time! Since I liked to cook a lot and build fires in our fireplace, I thought human hair might be the better choice. Knowing that I may be without hair for a year or so, my husband told me to make an appointment and see what I thought about this wig maker. We knew it was going to be relatively expensive, but given the length of time I was going to be wearing a wig; we decided it would be worth it.

The wig maker was named Piny, and his salon was in Beverly Hills. I checked out their website and then called. I ended up speaking directly to Piny himself and knew right away that this was the place for me. He was so warm and caring on the phone. He told me that he discounted wigs for cancer patients and couldn't wait to meet me. I knew from his website that he worked with many movie stars, but he treated me as though I was just the same as any one of them!

I made an appointment for the following week and Cheryl flew to Santa Barbara so she could drive to Beverly Hills with me—it was a fun twin day! Piny took all sorts of measurements of my head and asked me lots of questions like how long did I want it, what color, etc. I had long hair, but said shoulder length would be good and that I'd like my naturally dark blond color with highlights. At that time, my hair had gotten so thin and the color had become so blond that I was even thinking about getting low lights. He totally agreed and told me I needed darker hair to give it some dimension. He just said he would come up with the perfect color and hairstyle for me. I trusted that he knew what he was talking about and left very excited. By this time my hair had thinned out so much that it was barely holding on the fall.

It would be ten days before my new wig was going to be ready and I could hardly wait. Piny had another salon in Sherman Oaks, which is closer to Santa Barbara, so we arranged to meet him there to pick up the wig. My husband came with me that day and we were both totally blown away. The style and color were perfect for me and actually took years off my appearance because it was so youthful! I know that seeing the wig helped when he had to shave what little of my hair remained. I was told to wash the wig with regular shampoo, and they gave me a stand and foam head that I would need to blow dry the hair and style it. I had been told in the past that a human hair wig is harder to take care of, but for me it was very easy. After washing it and blowing it dry with round brushes, all I have to do is brush it every morning, and that's about it. If someone has some hair left on their head, they can use clips to secure a wig. But when you're bald, two-sided tape works great. I have been out in a windstorm with mine and it doesn't even budge. I just put it on, and out the door I go!

I know that not everyone likes to wear a wig—especially in the summer. Some people prefer to go bald, while others enjoy buying lots of different hats and scarves. But I love wearing a wig so that when I look in the mirror I see this healthy-looking person staring back at me. I think that one of the main things behind my positive attitude is feeling that cancer does not define me, but is just a disease that I need to deal with. Part of being able to feel that I'm going to beat the odds is looking healthy so that I can feel healthy. When I wake up in the morning and see this bald head with no eyebrows and no eyelashes, I feel differently. But when I put on the wig and some eyeliner, and pencil on some eyebrows, I totally feel like I can beat this disease. A common expression is *"fake it til you make it"* and maybe that's what I'm doing! Believe me, I've had some interesting emails on this topic (and most cancer patients have heard it all), saying things like, "hair is the least of your problems…it will grow back…it's a vanity thing…and a woman should just go out in public and feel proud being bald because beauty comes from within." I agree that beauty is from within, but that's not the point. It's great if someone chooses to go bald instead of wear a wig, or to wear a hat or a scarf. But if a person chooses to wear a wig, that should be fine too! None of us handle our cancer and the side effects of the drugs in exactly the same way. That's just natural— we're different people emotionally and physically. A person who has lost their hair, eyebrows, or eyelashes shouldn't feel guilty because they fall apart and cry when they see themselves in a mirror. It's a reminder that cancer is lingering in the body, and that to kill it we sometimes have to use harsh chemicals, which can damage healthy organs as well. It's also an emotional thing to lose one's identity and a woman's hair is part of her identity—at least it is for me!

When I lost my eyebrows and eyelashes along with my hair, it was a big change for me. The first time I lost my hair, my eyebrows and eyelashes stayed around. Eyelashes serve a practical purpose of protecting your eyes. Without them, my eyes became more sensitive. I didn't want to wear false eyelashes, but thought that putting on dark eyeliner would make a difference. It did. I recently spoke with someone in the chemo room that told me losing her hair wasn't as devastating for her as losing her eyelashes—I know what she means because your eyes seem to appear smaller—eyelashes tend to open up the eyes.

When I was at a local beauty supply shop they told me I should try a new product they had just gotten in called RevitaLash. It was created by Dr. Michael Brinkenhoff as a special gift to his wife while she was recovering from breast cancer. On his website he explained that her beautiful eyelashes had been damaged due to intensive chemotherapy. Dr. Brinkenhoff formulated an eyelash conditioner that he said, after just a few weeks, gave a renewed look of vitality to his wife's eyelashes. The box also had a statement that a portion of all proceeds benefit breast cancer research initiatives. So I bought the product.

But, when I got home and read the instruction sheet inside the box, I saw it said not to use RevitaLash if you are currently going through chemotherapy. I sent Dr. Brinkenhoff an email to ask about it. He wanted more information, including how often I was receiving Abraxane. He said, "In general, while a patient is actively on chemotherapy agents, I advise against using RevitaLash; however, there are exceptions." He suggested that since I actually lived close to his office, he would be happy to see me and give me his medical opinion. He went on to say "I know how important it can be to regain your lashes after they have been lost to chemotherapy and I would like to help, if I can."

When we met, he explained why it wouldn't be a good idea to use the product during chemotherapy. RevitaLash stimulated cells to grow new eyelashes, and chemotherapy specifically attacks fast-growing cells. That made perfect sense to me. If I used RevitaLash, the Abraxane would go directly to those fast-growing cells and kill them. So, the product wouldn't work anyway. I wanted Abraxane to concentrate on the tumors in the liver, not on my eyelashes! I appreciated the time Dr. Brinkenhoff took to meet with me—he really was very caring. I will save the product to use when I'm no longer on chemotherapy. And, in remission it will help me grow longer, thicker and fuller eyelashes! In the meantime, black eyeliner pencil does the trick, and a blond eyebrow pencil helps me create natural looking eyebrows.

In November 2006, a CT scan showed that there was "diminution of the extensive metastatic disease in the liver." The report also said there was improvement in the appearance of the liver and the exophytic mass that went from the liver to the peripancreatic region had diminished in size and that the spleen was normal and unchanged. WOW, this was the first good news in a very, very long time. I nearly screamed with delight when I saw those words on the page! My CA15-3 was also going in the right direction—down to 1080. It looked like Abraxane was working!

"It is reasonable to expect the doctor to recognize that science may not have all the answers to problems of health and healing."

—NORMAN COUSINS

CHAPTER ELEVEN

Rejecting the Prognosis

When I saw him in Los Angeles in September, Dr. Lapraz told he would not be able to make the trip to Idaho in December and asked if we could come to Paris instead. He felt it was important to see me every three months during this critical time. I knew that Abraxane could be given in a higher dose, which was administered once every three weeks, but that Dr. Woliver preferred I get it weekly. In order to make the trip to Paris possible, I asked if I could get the higher dose of Abraxane on a one-time basis in December. I would then follow it up with a Neulasta shot so I wouldn't have to worry about my white count being compromised during the trip. Dr. Woliver thought this would be workable, depending on how my blood tests looked. I went ahead and planned the trip as though everything would be just fine. Cheryl and Len decided to join Michael and me as well.

In the months before our trip, I had been experiencing a great deal of pain in my right knee. Dr. Woliver ordered an MRI so we could be sure that the cancer hadn't metastasized to bones in my leg. Right after the MRI, he emailed me with the good news that it wasn't cancer. However, the MRI had shown that I was experiencing all that pain because of severe damage to the cartilage and ligaments in my knee. His email to me said:

"your knee shows extensive degenerative tear of the anterior horn and body of the lateral meniscus, degeneration of the anterior cruciate ligament (but no tear), joint effusion, a large popliteal cyst, and a 'moderate' chondromalacia of the patella…whew, you must have been having fun! Time for you to see the knee surgeon when you return from France."

He gave me a prescription for an anti-inflammatory called Mobic. That helped with the pain and off we went to Paris!

We were so excited. I hadn't been to Paris since May 2005, and Michael and I hadn't been there together since December 2004. We were only going to be there for a week, but that would give us plenty of time to see new art exhibitions and dine at some of our favorite restaurants, in addition to keeping our appointments with Dr. Lapraz. When we got to our first appointment, there was another medical doctor present. He was from the Pasteur Institute, and Dr. Lapraz had been discussing my case with him. They asked if it would be all right for him to sit in during the exam. I said there would be no problem. His English was excellent and he had a wonderful bedside manner—I liked him immediately. They both discussed my blood work and talked about what the physical exam had shown. They seemed to agree that Abraxane was doing what it was supposed to, and that their job would be to help prolong the efficacy of the Abraxane, which they expected I would be on for around two years. After the doctor from the Pasteur Institute said his goodbyes, Cheryl, Len and Michael had their exams with Dr. Lapraz. They were all seeing him to bring their bodies into balance and prevent disease from occurring.

While in Paris, we saw our friends Patrice and Danny Pauly, as well as their daughter Gwénaëlle who had stayed with us for five months while interning at Michael's office. It was a great trip, but much too short!

Upon my return to Santa Barbara, I went back on a weekly chemo schedule. It was getting harder and harder for the chemo nurses to find a good vein for my infusions each week, and so one of the nurses told me it was time to get a port. Up until then, I had held off getting a port because I didn't know how long I would be on the Abraxane. And, if some new tablet form of chemo (like Sutent) were to become available, I might be going off Abraxane. I would then have to have another surgery to remove the port. But now it looked like Sutent wasn't in the near future, and I agreed that getting a port made sense. At the time I was pretty negative about going through the surgery to have the port put in, but in hindsight, I would have to say that it was definitely a good move. I might have been able to put it off for another month, but I hoped to have continued success with Abraxane for at least a year and maybe two. Putting off getting a port that long would have been out of the question.

The surgery for the port was outpatient and only took a couple of hours. I had something called a Power Port installed. It is the same size as a regular port, but it can also be used for the injection of contrast during a CT scan—something you can't do with a regular port. The BARD PowerPort, which is what I had put in, can withstand the power injector used for CT scans. I had a few days of discomfort around the site where the port was put in, but that quickly passed. Other than that, there have been no problems with the port and it has functioned flawlessly.

After the port was put in, I received a packet of information that included a PowerLoc Safety Infusion Set that would be necessary if I wanted to have my port used for a CT scan. The PowerPort system is only power injectable when accessed with a PowerLoc Safety Infusion Set. The next time I went in for a CT scan in February 2007, I showed this information to the technician. She was surprised to hear there was a port that could be used for a CT scan. She Xeroxed the information to show to other people at the lab. I didn't need them to use the port for my scan since they never have a problem accessing my veins. She also told me that at their lab only a radiologist or a registered nurse would be certified to access a port. Since there were no registered nurses working there they would have had to call a radiologist if I wanted them to use the port. She also mentioned if a radiologist had to start the scan, it would cost more money!

Once again, the news was good—the tumors in the liver had reduced in size and there were no new ones! The report said "Overall, particularly over the recent series of examinations, between July 2006 and the current study, there has been continuous diminution of the size of the lesions." Dr. Lapraz was going to be in Pocatello that month to give a seminar and to see patients. Off I went with the CT scan results and a new series of blood tests showing that my CA15-3 had gone down slightly to 633, the CA19-9 had also come down, and all my liver enzymes were in the normal range. This meant the Abraxane was continuing to do its job. Dr. Lapraz said I was definitely improving and that he was very pleased with the results he was following. He told me that Abraxane and the plant-based medicines he had prescribed for me were working together. He added that the tumors were being targeted while the rest of my organs were being protected. Besides helping to keep my body in balance, the endobiogenic medicines were helping me avoid many of the side effects of Abraxane, such as neuropathy and lack of energy. Another side effect I get from Abraxane is flushed cheeks, but just for a day or two following treatment.

On the airplane going home from Pocatello, a woman sitting next to me was reading a book called *The Secret*. I noticed it and asked her about it because I had recently heard a lot about the book. She told me that it was about positive thinking. When I got home, my sister Nancy called me to say she had just gotten this same book and that it was amazing. She suggested I read it. When things like this happen, I think they are messages for me, so I went to my favorite bookstore and bought a copy. Like any book, there may be parts you don't totally agree with, but overall, I liked the essence of its message. It wasn't really saying anything new, but it contained some wonderful examples of what positive thinking can accomplish. When I was in business I used to listen to motivational tapes by a speaker named Brian Tracy, and I thought the ideas expressed in *The Secret* were very similar.

One thing I got out of *The Secret* was to meditate on everything I had to be grateful for. I started doing it when going to bed every night. It would relax me and put me right to sleep before I even had a chance to get to all the people I'm so blessed to have in my life...like my amazing husband, my loving twin Cheryl, and sister Nancy, my brother Vernon, my children Michael, Kim and David, and my daughter-in-law Lisa, my dogs, my incredible team of doctors...the list goes on and on! I also try to wake every morning with my gratitude list. It starts my day on a positive note! Another tool I got from the book was how to immediately change your mood when you're feeling down or negative. For me, it was thinking about something that could put a smile on my face...like my little dog Mattie, or the day I got married and felt like a real princess, or actually just the thought of Ellen DeGeneres makes me laugh! These are little triggers that can instantly change a mood, and that was a gift *The Secret* gave me!

In March 2007, I had a bit of a scare. I began to have a pain on the left side of my rib cage where there had been a tumor in February 2000. We quickly scheduled a bone scan, and it was negative. Then a PET scan was ordered to be sure everything else was fine. At first the radiologist reading the PET scan said that the liver was "unremarkable." This meant that the scan didn't show cancer in the liver, and that just didn't make any sense! So Dr. Woliver had another radiologist read the scan. That doctor said that yes, there was activity in the liver, and that he couldn't rule out bone marrow involvement. This was very confusing and unsettling! Dr. Woliver said I could have a bone marrow biopsy as a follow-up test, but I didn't think that was necessary because my LDH was in the normal range and I knew that it would be high if there were bone marrow involvement. He agreed with me that it could be a false positive.

I made an appointment to see the PET scan myself and to talk with the radiologist who had written the second report. When I looked at the scan I didn't see anything that jumped out at me. The radiologist explained that he couldn't rule out bone marrow involvement because the scan showed a diffuse glow in the spine and ribs. He continued to say that he understood I hadn't had any Neupogen or Neulasta injections for many months. Those drugs would have thrown the test off. I told him that what he understood was completely wrong, and that I had had nine Neupogen shots every month for the past six months—including one the day before the PET scan. He was startled and apologized profusely. He said he would never have written that report had he known this, that it was a miscommunication, and that he now was certain there was no bone marrow involvement! This is just another example of why I believe so strongly that each patient must be the manager of his or her own disease. It's imperative that we as patients take an active role in our treatment.

Around this time, I emailed Dr. Woliver about adding the targeted-therapy drug Avastin (Bevacizumab) to my protocol. It was the first FDA approved biological therapy designed to inhibit the formation of new blood vessels to a tumor. He replied saying he thought Avastin would be great for me, but that he didn't think that my insurance company would approve it since it was still not FDA approved for breast cancer. Avastin had been FDA approved for the treatment of colorectal and lung cancers a few years ago, but was still in clinical trials (which had been very positive) for breast cancer.

Nevertheless, I knew of several breast cancer patients with metastases in their liver who were on a combination of Abraxane and Avastin, and it was proving to be very effective. A young woman in Maine told me that her insurance company would approve Avastin only if it was given in combination with a taxane like Abraxane, Taxol or Taxotere; which are drugs that kill cancer cells by stopping their growth. I had heard the same thing from other cancer patients. So I asked Dr. Woliver to please apply for it with my insurance company anyway, just so we could see what they said. In the meantime, I meditated and visualized about being in the chemo room and the nurse was putting up a bag of Avastin as part of my treatment. It was so real to me that I wasn't surprised a week later when I got a message on our answering machine from one of the chemo nurses telling me I would be in the chemo room an extra 90 minutes that week because Avastin was being added to my protocol. This sort of positive visualization was another gift from the book *The Secret!*

During my appointment with Dr. Woliver prior to the first infusion of Avastin, we talked about its side effects. He said mild nose bleeds or blood in the nose was common. He told me it was due to the conglomeration of superficial vessels that lie under the skin/mucosa of the nasal septae. Known as "Kiesselbach's triangle" (or Little's area), it is richly supplied with capillaries. They seem to be quite dependent on vascular endothelial growth factor (VEGF) to maintain their integrity. Blocking VEGF causes them to bleed more easily and Avastin is an anti VEGF therapy. According to recent research, VEGF is expressed in a variety of breast cancer types and is involved throughout the breast tumor life cycle. Dr. Woliver also mentioned that Avastin could cause complications with the healing of wounds, so any surgery would be unadvised while I was on the drug. That didn't seem to be a problem because I wasn't planning on having any surgery. But, I promptly told Dr. Woliver that actually I had been having a small amount of blood come out whenever I blew my nose ever since I started on Abraxane. I thought my nose was overly dry from having the heat on in our house. So, it's a nuisance to have the dry nose with blood, but it also means the Avastin is doing what it's supposed to be doing! I'd heard that using a saline nose spray three times a day could help, so I tried it and it worked. I also put a little Vaseline in each of my nostrils to keep them moist, and that has helped. After Avastin was added to my treatments every other week, all the tumor markers on my blood test came down drastically. It was an indication that Avastin was working well in conjunction with Abraxane.

As I have mentioned, an MRI done in December showed extensive damage in my right knee, including a torn meniscus. But since I was on Abraxane and Avastin, there could be no surgery to repair it, as there would be problems with healing. I didn't want to have surgery anyway, because the stress it would place on my body could activate the tumors in my liver even more! When Dr. Woliver asked how my knee was doing I told him I was experiencing a constant pain in my right shin. He told me that this pain was probably radiating from my knee. Since it appeared to be a nerve pain, I tried taking some Neurontin, a drug that I had been given some time earlier when we thought I had shingles. Neurotin stopped the pain in my shin! Dr. Woliver said that was wonderful, and when I told him I also wanted to see an acupuncturist, he referred me to Dr. Kathleen Zisser, a medical doctor who had specialized in physical medicine and rehabilitation before getting certified as an acupuncturist through a program for physicians at UCLA Medical School. She sounded like exactly what I needed.

I made an appointment with Dr. Zisser for later that week. I had been to an acupuncturist before, so I knew what to expect regarding the needles and how they were inserted. It amazed me to think back at how fearful I had once been when just looking at a needle. Now I was giving myself daily injections of mistletoe and starting acupuncture. I could hardly believe it! I remember watching television shows and cringed when I saw someone being treated with acupuncture, but there's really very little pain involved. Within a month, my knee was functioning at an almost normal and pain-free level. But, more importantly, Dr. Zisser was helping my body fight the cancer and working to counteract some of the side effects of Abraxane.

At my first appointment, Dr. Zisser took my history and examined me. She then asked me if I was feeling any tightness under my ribs. I had indeed been feeling tightness in my upper abdomen just below my ribs ever since I started on the Abraxane. I had just become so used to the sensation that I hadn't mentioned it to her. It almost feels like wearing a girdle high up under the breasts. She explained that in Chinese medicine this area is known as the hypochrondrium, and that it becomes symptomatic with liver problems. She explained that in her view, while chemo is necessary for advanced breast cancer, it also throws some of the body's systems out of balance. Chinese acupuncture attempts to re-establish that balance. She said acupuncture could help not only with the side effects of the chemotherapy, but also enhance the body's ability to fight the cancer by stimulating the immune system. In theory it is very similar to what Dr. Lapraz believes about getting the body back into balance.

Dr. Zisser went on to explain that when the needles are inserted into the body, the body gets the message and increases the flow of "Qi" (vital energy) and blood to the area. I noticed that when she inserted a needle in the area between my big toe and second toe, I felt a strong sensation. She explained that this point reflected an imbalance in my liver function. I also noticed that when a needle was inserted into the inside bend of my elbow and twirled, I again felt a strong sensation. She said this indicated I had a blockage in my intestines. I told her that I had just had chemo, and I get constipated from it. I came to understand that when you feel stimulation from a needle, it usually indicates a blockage of some sort. Think of a river that is blocked so that the water can't flow down to where it normally would go. By unblocking the channel, blood and Qi (vital energy) can flow through our bodies as they should. Acupuncture stimulates specific points on the body where energy collects and flows through pathways that are known as meridians and channels. They regulate the overall flow of energy and, therefore, allow the body to return to a state of balance and health. Dr. Zisser explained that acupuncture treatments are individually tailored for each patient, much like endobiogénie. It has been amazing to learn how acupuncture can help me with something as straightforward as pain in my knee, while at the same time helping my body get into balance to better fight cancer. Dr. Zisser was added to my gratitude list.

About this time, my twin sister had scheduled knee replacement surgery for her right knee. She also had a torn meniscus and other damage, which resulted in extremely painful bone-on-bone contact because no cartilage was left. We had both been athletic in high school and college, playing on the tennis team and involved with contemporary dance and gymnastics. It took a big toll on our knees. Cheryl arranged her surgery to be during my week off chemo so I could fly to Tucson and be with her. She was lucky to have a surgeon who did a gender-specific knee replacement, and kept the surgery minimally invasive by not cutting the quad muscle. That made rehabilitation much faster and easier.

Before I flew to Tucson, Dr. Zisser told me about a good meditation tape that she thought had been recorded by Norman Cousins, a prominent journalist, author and professor. She thought it would help Cheryl with her recovery. I couldn't find it at my local bookstore, and a search on their computer found no mention of it. But the store did have two of Norman Cousins' books in stock, and so I bought them. Again, things work out the way they're supposed to. Those books were exactly what I needed to read!

The first one was *Anatomy of an Illness as Perceived by the Patient*. I asked my husband if he had heard of Norman Cousins and he said "Yes, wasn't he the one who cured his debilitating disease through laughter?" I had heard many times that laughter can cure disease, but didn't associate the name of any particular person with the idea. I remembered that in the book, *The Secret*, they mentioned a woman who was inspired to include laughter as part of her healing after learning about the story of Norman Cousins. They stated in *The Secret:*

> "Norman had been diagnosed with an 'incurable' disease. The doctors told him he had just a few months to live. Norman decided to heal himself. For three months all he did was watch funny movies and laugh, laugh, laugh. The disease left his body in those three months, and the doctors proclaimed his recovery a miracle. As he laughed, Norman released all negativity, and he released the disease. Laughter really is the best medicine."

I agree that laughter is great for anyone with a disease, but after reading Norman Cousins' book I discovered that laughter wasn't exactly what cured his illness—popular folklore aside.

In reading *Anatomy of an Illness,* I learned that in 1964 Norman Cousins had been diagnosed with a serious collagen illness—a disease of the connective tissue, similar to arthritic and rheumatic diseases. He was told that a specialist who had consulted on his case put his chances for full recovery at one in five hundred. This specialist had also said he'd never personally witnessed a recovery from someone in these circumstances. That was when Cousins decided that if he was to be that "one in five hundred" he was going to have to be something much more than just a passive observer of his treatment.

Cousins knew that in order to combat severe arthritis it was important to get his endocrine system functioning fully—particularly the adrenal glands. First, he thought about the pain relieving and anti-inflammatory medications he was taking—drugs like aspirin and phenylbutazone. He learned that these drugs put a heavy load on the adrenal glands. He knew that going off these drugs would mean a great deal of pain, but he felt that he could live with it if he knew that progress was being made. He had read in the medical press that vitamin C helps to oxygenate the blood and that many people suffering from collagen diseases are deficient in vitamin C.

This was when he started thinking that vitamin C may play a vital role in feeding the adrenal glands and decided to discuss this with his doctor. The wonderful thing was that his doctor listened to him and was willing to set aside powerful drugs when he became convinced that his patient might have something better to offer. His doctor was wise enough to understand that the will to live is essential to recovery. He felt that it was important for Cousins to continue to believe that vitamin C was helping with his disease and improving the possibilities of recovery.

While Cousins was still being treated in the hospital, he first realized that laughter could help with his pain. He had a projector and some Marx Brothers movies brought into his room. He discovered that ten minutes of genuine belly laughter had an anesthetic effect that would give him at least two hours of pain-free sleep. When the pain-killing effect of the laughter wore off, he would have the projector turned back on and, more often than not, it would lead to another pain free sleep interval. He also discovered that a decrease in pain gave him a corresponding increase in mobility. Many years later he learned that laughter probably played a part in activating the release of endorphins.

The laughter was becoming a problem at the hospital, but soon he left and moved into a hotel, under the supervision of his doctor and with a nurse to give him high doses of vitamin C intravenously. This is what he believed actually cured his disease. He kept watching funny movies to help with the pain and to boost his immune system. After eight days of this routine, Cousins was able to move his thumbs without pain. This was when he had no doubt that he would make a full recovery. It took months before he could reach for a book on a high shelf, but year-by-year his mobility improved and he was basically pain free except for one shoulder and both knees. He was able to walk without the use of metal braces, and got back to playing tennis and golf.

A full seven years after the onset of his illness, he read in a medical journal that there was scientific confirmation of the dangers of using aspirin in the treatment of collagen diseases. The study pointed out how aspirin could be antagonistic to the retention of vitamin C in the body and that patients with rheumatoid arthritis should be taking vitamin C supplements, since it had been noted that most of them were deficient in vitamin C.

Norman Cousins writes that it is important to point out that he didn't regard the use of laughter as a substitute for traditional medical care. He also said that he tried to bring the full range of positive emotions into play—love, hope, faith, will to live, festivity, purpose, and determination. Cousins believed that the treatment of illness has to be carefully tailored to suit each individual patient. I bring this up because that's exactly what endobiogénie is all about—every patient has to be evaluated and treated individually!

When asked what he thought about having specialists tell him that his disease was progressive and incurable, Cousins said that "since he didn't accept the verdict, he wasn't trapped in the cycle of fear, depression and panic that frequently accompanies a supposedly incurable illness." Deep down, he knew that he had a good chance of recovery and liked the idea of beating the odds! I can so relate to this. When I was given a three percent chance of beating my cancer, I thought about the fact that actual people made up those three percent. So, why shouldn't I be one of them! I realized at that moment I would need to learn everything I could about breast cancer and the therapies there were available. I knew that the first step would be to stabilize the cancer. I honestly felt that I could live with cancer and treat it like a chronic condition—like diabetes or heart disease.

Ten years after he had been diagnosed with a supposedly incurable illness, Norman Cousins was walking down a street in New York City when he happened to meet one of the specialists who had given him the diagnosis of progressive paralysis. He immediately shook the doctor's hand with a very firm grip—so much so that the doctor had to let go because it was painful. The doctor could see that Cousins was fully recovered, and was eager to hear how it had come about. Cousins said, "It all began when I decided that some experts don't really know enough to make a pronouncement of doom on a human being." He ended the encounter by saying that he hoped doctors would be careful about what they said to others. "After all," he said, "they might be believed and that could be the beginning of the end.

After finishing the *Anatomy of an Illness,* I read another Norman Cousins book called *Head First: The Biology of Hope and the Healing Power of the Human Spirit.* It tells about his incredible work with UCLA's Program in Psychoneuroimmunology, which is a new branch of medicine based on the interaction of the brain, the endocrine system and the immune system. Everything I knew about Dr. Lapraz's work with endobiogénie is completely compatible with what Norman Cousins described in this book.

It's interesting to note that although Norman Cousins was not a medical doctor, he was an Adjunct Professor in the UCLA School of Medicine from 1978 until his death in 1990. He was also the first person to ever be awarded an honorary medical degree by the Yale University School of Medicine. He was a board member of the Harvard School of Public Health and the Institute for the Advancement of Health. Cousins had always maintained a deep interest in medical science and the human healing system, He even wrote about it from time to time in the *Saturday Review,* where he was editor from 1940-1971.

What interested me most about Cousins' work at UCLA was that he was able to prove that the mind plays a crucial role in a patient's ability to fight disease. It had been well established through previous research that we could make ourselves physically ill through negative emotions such as hate, fear, panic, depression, frustration, and despair. But the idea that positive emotions might actually help activate healing forces in the endocrine and immune systems had not been proven. Through research that he was involved in, and hundreds of interviews with doctors and patients, Cousins was able to show that an optimistic outlook and a strong relationship between patient and doctor increased a patient's chances of survival.

Throughout his book, Cousins makes it very clear that the cancer patients he observed who survived longer than others with the same disease did not deny their diagnosis, but they did deny and defy the verdict that was supposed to go with it! Those patients had a fierce determination to overcome their disease and beat the odds they had been given. Many people are surprised when they hear that cancer metastasized to my liver in 1999. I believe that the fact I look and feel so great in spite of all the treatments I've had to undergo is largely because I too accepted the diagnosis but not the prognosis!

After ten years at UCLA, Norman Cousins wrote a report for the Dean of the Medical School summarizing what he had experienced during a decade of working with patients and doctors. This is a portion of what his report said:

> "Few things I have learned in the past ten years have hit me more forcibly than the need of the physician to pay attention to the environment of treatment. What stood out most in the meetings I have had with more than 500 seriously ill patients over the years was that their condition deteriorated sharply at the time of the diagnosis. The moment they had a label to attach to their symptoms they became perceptibly worse. The label had certain connotations. These connotations led to panic, helplessness, and depression, all of which imposed psychological penalties—and

*all of which underlined the overriding importance of the physician's abil-
ity to communicate a diagnosis in a way that challenged but did not
crush the patient."*

*"Ten years ago, I thought that iatrogenic problems (those caused directly
by medical examination or treatment) were represented solely by physician error in the treatment of patients, i.e., mistakes in diagnosis or surgery or harmful effects of prescribed medications, etc. It became apparent to me over the years, however, that errors or failures in communica-
tion can be equally iatrogenic. The psychological devastation caused by
inartistically delivered diagnosis may be no less serious than mistakes in
medication or surgery. The doctor who gives a terminal date cannot be
absolutely certain in every case that his prediction is correct—yet that
prediction can have the effect of a hex and impair effective treatment."*

Cousins understood that physicians fear they could be at risk if something on the downside should occur that comes as a surprise to the
patient. But he pointed out that

*"It is also true that the patient who is emotionally crippled by the man-
ner of diagnosis is halfway down the hill before treatment even begins.
The emotional state in which the patient leaves the doctor's office can set
the stage for optimal treatment or for noncompliance, defeatism, and
depression."*

Many oncologists, unfortunately, still seem to be unaware of this simple yet vital concept. I know a breast cancer patient whose cancer has
metastasized to her liver, like mine. Her oncologist recently told her that
if she didn't respond to a new therapy, she would have only one to three
months to live. I couldn't even believe it! She told me that she made sure
her life insurance papers were in order, etc. She also mentioned that she
was surprised that she wasn't as devastated by the news as she thought
she would be. I was hoping that she wasn't accepting the prognosis,

because I knew that her liver enzyme levels were not much out of the normal range, and her tumor markers were also not that far from normal. There were still many therapies that were good options that she hadn't even tried. I was furious that her doctor had made this dire pronouncement and I let her know how I felt! My concern was that she would feel her life was over before even starting on the new protocol, and that it would affect how she responded to it.

When I was writing about her experiences for my book, I emailed her to be sure what I was saying was accurate. She told me:

> "You wrote my little story perfectly. I was in total shock after that appointment. YOUR email starting out 'First of all, your doctors are not God and can't give you that prognosis with any time attached!' really helped me. It made me hopeful. I was surprised when you said your liver enzymes had been much higher than mine and that you had been okay. I really needed to hear that. It changed how I looked at things. One example is when my daughter got her cell phone wet and we needed to get a replacement. Before your email I remember actually thinking that maybe I shouldn't buy her a new phone because she can just have mine in a month or so after I'm gone. Now THOSE kinds of thoughts are not going to help anyone's immune system! Fortunately I got her a new phone a few days later."

WOW! She really had accepted the doctor's prognosis! I honestly can't understand why doctors don't comprehend how much impact their words can have on a patient's mental attitude and their ability to fight their disease!

I think of another cancer survivor that I met on the Avon 3-Day Walk in 2000. Her oncologist had told her to go home and write her will. She chose not to believe the prognosis and went on to beat the odds. I met her ten years after her doctor had made that pronouncement! When doctors deliver this sort of programmed death sentence, it can become a self-ful-filling prophecy that serves to impair treatment. I can understand that an oncologist would need to say that the situation is serious and that a new course of treatment should be started immediately. But there is no reason that the oncologist could not add that many patients have responded very positively to this new protocol. Doctors don't have a crystal ball that tells them exactly what their patient's life expectancy is. What they are making is an educated guess, but it's still a guess! Thankfully, my oncologist doesn't believe in assigning survival times, because he doesn't feel a doctor knows for sure that will be the case. He takes an optimistic attitude about new treatments and backs it up with statements like "there are many other therapies we can still try, and new ones are con-stantly coming out of clinical trials." Hope is what every patient is look-ing for. It's the wise physician who works with the will to live and makes the hopes of the patient an integral part of the therapy, treating them as importantly as the medicines they prescribe.

Those of us dealing with breast cancer need to know that there are several very promising drugs currently in clinical trials. One chemother-apy drug called Ixabepilone has shown very good results with women who have not had success with such chemotherapies as anthracyclines (Adriamycin), taxanes (Taxol, Taxotere, Abraxane), and Xeloda. Research has also shown that Ixabepilone given with Xeloda increases the effec-tiveness of Xeloda. It's expected that this chemotherapy may become available by the end of 2007. There are also some very good new therapies for HER2+ breast cancer patients. In addition to the very effective Herceptin/Navelbene combination, there is a new targeted therapy called Tykerb, which was FDA approved in March 2007 to be given in conjunc-tion with Xeloda. A nice thing about Tykerb and Xeloda is that they are both in pill form—meaning no sitting in a chemo room! There are also other targeted agents similar to Avastin in the pipeline that promise to be even more effective. Just remember, the next new treatment on the horizon could be the one your body will respond to.

As I write this in September 2007 I am getting Abraxane and Avastin every other week, and they continue to work for me. In fact, my CA 15-3 tumor marker just came down from 570 to 445 (below 32 is the normal range for this lab). That was great news because it's the lowest my CA 15-3 has been since June 2006 when it was on the upward climb! My CA19-9 tumor marker is also down to the almost normal range, which it hasn't been since January 2006. This is a further indication of how well this combination of conventional treatment and endobiogenic medicines is working for me. How long it will continue to work is not something we know.

Wouldn't it be wonderful to know in advance which therapies would be most effective for each individual person? That might not be such a far-fetched concept. A friend of mine with fourth stage breast cancer recently went to a private clinic in Germany (the Leonardis Clinic) for an evaluation. She found it fascinating. They did a blood test called a "chemosensitivity test" where results indicate which chemotherapy or other therapy will be most effective for that particular person's tumor. She told me that the lab isolates the malignant cells in a blood sample, develops cell cultures, and then tests each culture with chemos and other cancer medicines that have already been approved or are in development. They also test the cultures with all sorts of other factors from co-enzyme 10 to various herbs in order to see what the malignant cells are sensitive to. It takes about ten days to get the results. I found this very interesting. I had originally heard of this clinic a year earlier from a journalist who was writing a review of my book. She had written an article about an American cancer patient who went there for an evaluation. That person had responded very well to the chemos suggested by the clinic's oncologists, who then worked as a team with the patient's oncologist back home. I hope that this type of testing will soon become available to cancer patients in United States.

I firmly believe that part of our job as patients is to accept a certain measure of responsibility for our own recovery. More than 2,000 years ago, a Roman philosopher named Seneca observed, "It is part of the cure to wish to be cured." He also believed that any length of life is sufficient if lived wisely. Our will to live and maintain a positive attitude in the face of a difficult diagnosis will make the outcome that much better. Certainly, being diagnosed with cancer would fill anyone with fear. But that kind of fear can put a stranglehold on one's actions and make it impossible for him or her to move forward. It's important to conquer the fear and replace it with hope. If an individual can stay positive and have confidence that their disease can be stabilized, whatever years they have left will be much more fulfilling. And, who could ask for more—regardless of the state of their health?

I recently heard an amazing interview by David Gregory (NBC's Chief White House Correspondent) with Tony Snow, who was then the White House Press Secretary. They spoke about Snow's battle with colon cancer. In summarizing what Snow had been saying, Gregory made this profound statement: "The lesson is don't withdraw into the disease." Snow quickly added, "Then it wins!" Tony Snow also mentioned that we forget what we have when we don't have something like this illness to deal with—I think it's a wake-up call. Living with something like advanced breast cancer is an on-going battle, but one needs to have confidence that it can be stabilized. It is also important to take the time to live life to its fullest and appreciate what we do have.

One of the first things I did when the cancer metastasized in my liver over seven years ago was to get a new puppy. That was when Mattie came into our lives. She has continued to make my life so full of laughter and love. We recently decided it was time to get another new puppy, and therefore, an adorable dark silver standard poodle puppy named Otis has become part of our family. It's so much fun to watch Otis and Mattie chase each other around the house and yard. Otis is at that stage where he's growing tall and he's so awkward that you just can't help but laugh when he stumbles down some stairs or grabs hold of the bathroom tissue and runs down the hall thinking this is the greatest fun! Poor Katie, our 13-year-old Lab, has to put up with Otis jumping all over her and tugging at her ears. What a good sport she is! I have found that having a puppy is such a great way to get completely away from cancer!

My battle with cancer has been a life-changing journey, and I've learned many things along the way. I've come to realize that a person needs to be proactive when deciding which treatments to pursue, and that they should be open to new and complementary therapies. I've also learned that many things can throw your body out of balance, that it takes work to get it back into balance, and that it's all just a part of living life. Today, I feel great and, for the most part, free of stress. I now know that my work did not define me. I have come to understand how stress can affect one's health. Finding the correct balance between work, family, and personal time is absolutely vital in lowering stress and creating harmony within. Maintaining a positive attitude has also been an integral part of my therapy. When I was first diagnosed, there were many things I wondered if I would be around to watch happen. But I chose to live life as though I would. Recently I was lucky to experience the joy of having my daughter Kim receive a graduate degree from New York University! Now I am concentrating on seeing my grandchildren being born! I hope that others can learn to bring their bodies into balance as I have, and treat their cancer as a chronic illness—without fear, but with hope.

The next chapter includes excerpts from an upcoming book by Drs. Lapraz and Duraffourd that explains endobiogénie. They gave me authorization to publish this material so that readers would have a better understanding of endobiogénie and how it has helped in my battle with cancer. While parts of it may be somewhat technical, it's well worth the read!

"Research is to see what everybody else has seen and to think what nobody else has thought."

— ALBERT SZENT-GYÖRGYI

CHAPTER TWELVE

Endobiogénie and Its Application to Cancer

WRITTEN BY CHRISTIAN DURAFFOURD, M.D.
AND JEAN-CLAUDE LAPRAZ, M.D.

TRANSLATED FROM THE FRENCH BY PATRICE PAULY AND COLIN NICHOLLS

A preliminary note from Carol Silverander:

I chose to write a book about living with Stage Four breast cancer so that others who find themselves in a similar situation might benefit from what I've learned. I hope the knowledge I've gained will help guide them through the difficult choices they face, and assist them in achieving the best possible outcome.

Toward that end, I want my readers to be able to take full advantage of everything that I have experienced. Undoubtedly, one of my most valuable experiences has been a complementary form of treatment called endobiogénie that I have received from two physicians in Paris, France. Endobiogénie is a new, all-encompassing approach to medicine that was conceived by Dr. Christian Duraffourd and developed with Dr. Jean-Claude Lapraz over the past several decades. They each have more than 30 years of experience as physicians, including seven years in the Department of General Surgery and Oncology at Boucicaut Hospital in Paris.

I am, therefore, devoting this final chapter to a more complete explanation of the endobiogenic approach to medicine, as practiced by Drs. Duraffourd and Lapraz. In this chapter, which is excerpted from a book they will soon publish, they explain how and why endobiogénie works, and discuss the promise it holds for dealing with all types of medical problems. It's a fascinating story, and one that's well worth reading and remembering.

This chapter also includes a visit-by-visit record of my appointments with Dr. Lapraz. It shows, in some detail, how endobiogénie was applied—quite effectively, I might add—to my cancer. Dr. Lapraz and my friend, Patrice Pauly, have been instrumental in helping me better understand many of the rather complex concepts involved. Here, then, is what the doctors have written.

An Introduction to Endobiogénie

Throughout history, impressive advances have been made in understanding the physical, chemical and biological functions of the human body and the mechanisms of disease. In modern times, research steadily narrowed its focus from the body as a whole to the separate organs. Then the focus went from organs to tissues, tissues to cells, and finally to the individual components that make up each cell. Today, many scientists pin their hopes on the work being done with the smallest known unit of information, the gene. Billions of dollars ride on the expectation that gene therapy will one day provide an effective treatment for all diseases.

This approach to medicine, which we will refer to as the "reductionist approach," was sparked many years ago by the discovery of germs and the ways in which they relate to infectious diseases. The germ was seen as the root cause of disease and it was thought that its destruction would resolve all problems. This approach dictates that finding an efficient antibiotic would cure the disease, and that infectious diseases would eventually vanish from the earth. But now, after more than 50 years of over-consumption of antibiotics, the number of infectious diseases has not been reduced. Disease is not always cured through the use of antibiotics. Relapses have become more frequent, particularly when a disease is chronic and attacks someone who is weakened or debilitated. Germs develop their own defenses and we have seen the return of infectious diseases—such as tuberculosis—once thought to have been eliminated in developed countries.

A similar situation evolved with the reductionist approach to treating cancer. An abnormal cell was thought to be the root cause of the pathology, and it was believed that the destruction of the abnormal cells would cure the disease. Finding an efficient drug that would inhibit the division of cells seemed to be all that was needed. It was commonly thought that the discovery of the right drug could eradicate cancer in just a few decades. Unfortunately, the reality of the situation turned out to be quite different. While short-term survival rates did improve, the number of relapses and metastases increased. Now, the number of new cancers has surged to such a level that it is predicted that one out of three children born after the year 2000 will suffer from some type of cancer during their lifetime.

How can we explain, not so much these failures, but the inability to predict them? One reason is that the reductionist approach to medicine assumes the existence of some outside inducing agent—such as a germ—for any pathology. This approach focuses only on symptoms, and never deals with the host. It does not consider the global functioning of the human body—a complex mechanism in which all elements are interdependent and linked to one another.

Each of these elements plays a role, according to clearly defined rules, in order to keep the system in balance—even if maintaining this balance involves the appearance of a disease. A disease, therefore, reflects the difficulties encountered by the organism in maintaining balance. It is the cost of this maintenance, and also the cost to the organism, of having given up part of its "territory."

This internal regulatory process creates the conditions that allow a pathological state (or disease) to exist, emerge and persist. A disease is rarely caused solely by an external aggressor, physical trauma, or overwhelming contagion. The aggressor generally plays nothing more than a triggering role. Endobiogénie explains how this system functions.

What is Endobiogénie?

The theory of endobiogénie is based upon the concept that the human organism functions internally as a cohesive unit, and the theory lays down rules for this functioning.

Endobiogénie can be defined as the fundamental expression of the potential capacities of a living being, based on his or her genetic inheritance and its fusion into a certain initial physical state that provides that individual's touchstone of physiological equilibrium. It gives priority to:

- The role of the host in relation to the illness, at each stage of the cohabitation of the two;
- The study of all the mechanisms that regulate the internal environment, both in itself and in relation to the external environment in which it lives;
- The study of everything that links and coordinates these mechanisms, and of everything that guarantees their smooth running and the maintenance of internal equilibrium.

The bodily system that assumes responsibility for all of this must necessarily be unique, unified, and ubiquitous. And it must be able permanently to govern the organism in its entirety. Only the endocrine system possesses all the qualities needed to carry out these functions. For it is the only bodily system that is present, or represented, everywhere simultaneously. Furthermore it is the only one to react and to respond to every demand of a physiological nature, whether such demands are internal—that is, endocrine—whether they participate in metabolism as a whole, or whether they are responding to stimuli from the sense organs.

The endocrine system alone is capable of preserving homeostatic stability (its physiological touchstone) and restoring the integrity of the organism whenever this is compromised.

Apart from this basic role of maintenance, and that of nutrition, the endocrine system also regulates the different developmental phases of life, from growth to "the finality of birth" (in scientist Jean Rostand's words), passing through the different stages of restructuring.

This will to maintain constant control over the internal balance of one's own system, as well as over that of homeostasis—the internal equilibrium of the whole organism—implies the existence of permanent compensatory mechanisms within the body. Whether they are synergistic or antagonistic, these phenomena of permanent auto-adaptation within the endocrine system express the reality of the endobiogenic environment. They represent our continuous internal struggle for life, and for quality of life, up until the point where the organism is forced to trade illness for survival. This latter appears to be an absurdity, but is in fact not so, because illness represents a last-ditch attempt by the organism to preserve its integrity.

The theory of endobiogénie, and its biological application—which is known as the Biology of Functions—scientifically demonstrates the existence of this defense process and its means of implementation. It also scientifically demonstrates:

- The essential fallacy of experimental medicine, originating with Claude Bernard—its permanent exclusion of the reality of the living being;

- The permanent failure of this approach's founding principle—the concept of one illness, one causal agent (whether internal or external);

- The limits (this applies to all sciences) of the binary system and the need to replace it by a ternary system, which alone can reflect the reality of life.

Each of our internal organization's functional units is based on the triad of action, reaction and regulation. Only such a mode of activity can allow the organism to achieve its ends with the necessary degree of precision—function by function, organ by organ, system by system. It is thus present, in a hierarchical manner, at every level of our organized global system.

Each of our internal organization's functional units is based on the triad of action, reaction and regulation. Only such a mode of activity can allow the organism to achieve its ends with the necessary degree of precision—function by function, organ by organ, system by system. It is thus present, in a hierarchical manner, at every level of our organized global system.

As a structured system of protection, a disease follows the same set of rules. Because it is physiological before it becomes pathological, disease cannot be conceived of without the conjunction of the three elements that constitute the real causes of the pathology.

These three elements are absolutely necessary to the existence, maintenance and duration of the pathology. If one of these elements fails, falters, or is interrupted, this will be enough to hinder or block the process of manifestation of the disease. This is the case regardless of the intensity and the power of the external aggressor that is deemed to be the causative agent. As we have said, the organism is largely responsible for its own pathogenicity, and it is entirely responsible for its pathological manifestations:

- The first element of this triad is structural;

- The second element is also linked to structure and concerns what we have referred to above as auto-adaptation;

- The third element is purely adaptive and depends on the mechanism set up by the organism to fight aggression, whatever its type, intensity, or duration, however new it is to the organism, however often it has been repeated, and whatever the problems left over from past aggressions. This mechanism, even though it is relative like the other two, is key in that it determines the most suitable means, from an endobiogenic point of view, of self-healing—that is, the means that appears to the organism to be best adapted to survival, in that it matches as closely as possible the equilibrium associated with the organism's specific endobiogenic state, taking into account all information available.

To get the most efficient return—apart from in emergency cases—any external therapy must remain closely linked with and be least disturbing to the organism's regular operation. That is, the aggressivity of any treatment, which is linked both to the fact that it has to be digested (which is very onerous for the body) and to its action (which necessarily seeks to disrupt the system and therefore generates a reaction), must be less than the positive effect that is sought.

This implies that, before deciding on an in-depth treatment, the practitioner has to assess three things:

- The first concerns the illness itself—its diagnosis, its specific causes (etiology), how far and how fast it has developed, how invasive it is;
- The second concerns the patient him or herself—his current endobiogenic status, in terms of reactivity and adaptation, and the diagnosis of the causes of his pathology, (i.e. his basic endobiogenic structure), its step-by-step evolution up to the precritical and then critical phase of illness, and the speed of its progress;
- The third concerns the degree of coexistence between the patient and his pathology: the relative level of structural versus adaptational activities, and the dominance of one over the other.

Only when these three things have been determined will it be possible to decide what the priority should be:

- The direct reduction of the potential of the illness;

- Or support for the capacity of the organism to combat illness.

In all cases, an in-depth etio-endobiogenic treatment is required.

The follow-up treatment should be based on a continuing assessment of these three factors, and on the resulting evaluation of the therapeutic activity up to that point. Therefore, the therapeutic priority is to stop the process of degradation by first restoring the capacity of adaptation, moving from the superficial to the structural, until one manages to restore the capacity for auto-adaptation.

This means first getting back to a basal equilibrium before making any attempt to modify that equilibrium in order to definitively rule out any risk of a return to a crisis state. In other words, the therapeutic priority is to re-establish an appropriate balance between the proper interests of the patient and the means of expression of the illness—an illness to which the patient has conceded part of himself in order to reduce 'management costs' and to permit the maintenance of the remaining structure, which then can be better managed at less cost.

This triple assessment and its corollary, which is made possible only by an in-depth clinical examination, is based on a knowledge of the physiological data expressing the functionality of the organism. In order to facilitate this approach and demonstrate its scientific value in a quantifiable and reproducible way, a new tool of biological assessment has been created. That tool is the Biology of Functions.

The purpose of the Biology of Functions is to quantify the functional abilities of the organism, before and after the effects of adaptation. Because it is in permanent movement, functionality can only be measured by a dynamic, integrated and evolutionary methodology. Each function is quantified by an index, specified by a level of activity and qualified by a score. The index expresses the resulting effectiveness of its activity, both in itself and in relation to the metabolic tissular needs of the organism.

The whole set of indexes gives a very precise evolutive assessment of an individual body's functionality, system by system, organ by organ. These indexes are calculated mostly from commonly used blood analysis data using formulae that reflect the modalities of functionality. Reliability and reproducibility are provided by a computer-based model which simultaneously determines the whole set of indexes.

The Biology of Functions allows one to determine the pathogenic tendencies of the organism, the stage of development, and the degree of severity of a potential pathology. It can also be used as a tool to track the natural development of the pathology and its development under treatment, in order to better adjust the latter.

Choosing the Best Therapy

Apart from emergency situations, when the patient's life is at stake and risks must be accepted, the therapy must always provide a result no worse than the disease being treated. The risk of "the cure being worse than the disease" is particularly high in the case of long-term treatments, when side effects may not be apparent for some time.

However, prescription is an essential part of the medical act. Hippocrates' principle of 'primum non nocere' (above all, do no harm), was taken by us 20 years ago as a basis for the wider concept of 'essential non-harm,' which we adopted as a fundamental rule of medical practice. This principle is becoming increasingly neglected by modern medicine, which appears less and less adapted to long-term treatment. Whatever their objective—as a cure for chronic pathologies, as a palliative, or as a preventative—treatments based on the use of substitutive drugs appear, in the long term, to be more harmful than beneficial, because suppressing the illness will inevitably lead to it expressing itself in a different form, regardless of the nature or the origin of the remedy used.

This is why we created, some 30 years ago, the concept of clinical phytotherapy. Clinical phytotherapy is an approach that gives medicinal plants a prominent place in a therapeutic arsenal chosen for its capacity to satisfy this fundamental principle of "doing no harm." The term "clinical phytotherapy" in itself implies adherence to endobiogenic principles.

Like a patient, a medicinal plant needs to be considered in terms of its global structure and not of its individual constituents taken separately. A plant's multiple properties, taken as a whole, are geared to a specific end that is unique to that plant. This is because the plant possesses a coherence of action and reaction which limits its effects according to internal rules, comparable to those that govern our physiological regulation.

Therefore, there are two basic rules for the use of medicinal plants in endobiogenic treatment:

- Producers should aim to extract the full spectrum of active constituents from these plants;
- Practitioners should use only full-spectrum extracts in practice.

This kind of use of medicinal plants requires a profound knowledge of the plants' overall properties, and of their simultaneous and synergistic impact on the organism. Adherence to these rules will meet the requirements of clinical phytotherapy, in terms of:

- Guaranteeing an action of therapeutic induction that fully respects the patient's physiology and eschews any form of substitution;
- Using the individual and synergistic properties of medicinal plants to good effect in order to keep doses to a strict minimum, thus reducing the risk of effects that are adverse or the opposite of those desired.

Nutrition and Its Therapeutic Effect

Like any medication, food should not generate worse effects than the pathology itself. Cancer is an illness like any other. The development of cancer implies the contribution of a tissue or a set of tissues, an organ or a set of organs, associated with an increase in their manufacturing function, which is part of the adaptation process.

Once a certain production threshold has been passed, tissue restructuring occurs, aimed at increasing the size, volume, and the longevity of each production unit. One must therefore be careful not to encourage tumor growth by eating foods that provide, in a readily usable form, all the necessary ingredients for its expansion. This is true regardless of the stage of cancer development.

The supply of protein precursors accelerates and amplifies the work of production, which is the aim of this factory of war. Carbohydrates provide the energy supply, which is the fuel for the production cells' motor. Lipids guarantee the long-term energy supply, and provide the structural limits to this factory complex with its specific purpose.

One of the main characteristics of a tumor is its hyperadaptability, which is the very essence of its being. This is why the complete suppression of food, as in total and prolonged fasts, as well as certain mono diets, will have a spectacular effect, but if the real endobiogenic cause of the cancer is not eliminated, the tumor will start to expand again as soon as food is reintroduced. It will adapt its internal metabolism to any source of nutrition available. This is why we prefer to prescribe personalized diets, which can be adapted to the stage of development of the illness—or at most alternating mono diets—rather than full fasts.

The priority, therefore, is to reduce the overall work of the organism in order to allow it both to reduce its demand on this misdirected system of adaptation and to reduce its nutrition. It is most important to reduce the workload of the organs of elimination, particularly that of the liver and of its detoxifying function, in order to free it up to perform its endocrino-metabolic role.

The elimination of high-glycemic-index carbohydrates is an absolute priority, considering their role at every level of metabolism—particularly that of tumor cells, which eat their weight in glucose every four to five hours.

The elimination of dairy products is mandatory at all stages of the disease, particularly during the inflammatory phases, because they provide—in a decreasing order of concentration for cow's milk, goat's milk and (much less) sheep's milk—proteins that are precursors of inflammatory proteins.

Finally, animal proteins should be eliminated during phases in which the tumor is rapidly developing, because such proteins are infinitely more easily assimilated by the organism and are a delicacy for tumor cells, which delight in them. This is why, if patients are unable totally to give up red meat, fish and poultry should be recommended since they are less immediately toxic. In general, one should recommend the following foods:

- Vegetables (raw and cooked);
- Fruits (preferably uncooked);
- Vegetables rich in fiber (all bran cereals, beans), calcium (broccoli) and magnesium (spinach, corn);
- Fruit monodiets (grapes, melon, red fruits).

Endobiogénie and Cancer

As stated above, cancer is a particular method of adaptation by the organism, which, as such, follows completely endobiogenic rules. Its evolution and its manifestations are most often an expression of the organism's responses to external aggressions. This explains the link, often wrongly made, between symptoms and an assumed agent.

As for any pathology, it is necessary to determine the route followed by the organism in bringing about such a situation and to reduce both the needs engendered by this situation and its ability to express itself. As with any restructuring process, the required treatment regime is a lengthy business, in which the role of the patient is critical, both in terms of his or her full adherence to the regime and in making the necessary efforts to take their life in hand, and tame their illness. It is essential that this requirement is fully understood.

Better than any long explanation, the endobiogenic account of how Carol's cancer arose illustrates the way in which an illness is generated by the organism itself. Endobiogénie teaches us that our life is punctuated by phases of restructuring that allow the organism to actively remove bad physiological "habits" and blockages, such as toxic states, which have built up since the last phase of restructuring.

Carol was 41 years old when she began the major phase of restructuring that allows the organism to prepare for menopause. She already possessed a structure with a fundamentally very active gonadotropic axis, with a clear hyper-estrogenic state, even a hyperfolliculinic state. She also had an overactive thyroid axis centered on the pairing TRH-thyroid. This association simultaneously increases glucidic and insulinic activity and multiplies intracellular activity and protein production. It requires a major increase in inflammatory activity to raise both the intracellular concentration of nutrient transporters and tissular congestion to allow their development, and thus assure an increase in the compensatory production of estrogen receptors.

All this requires the activation of the corticotropic axis to allow the normal restructuring process to be definitively put into action and to guarantee that aromatization (a process which converts androgens into estrogens) takes place.

This specific hormonal environment targets a number of tissues rich in estrogen receptors. These are located in the breast, and more specifically in the left breast and more actively in the upper quadrants, and also in the left lobe of the liver, and the bones. The thyroid context here reduces the risk of cerebral metastases that would normally be present with this type of endobiogenic equilibrium in which pancreatic activity has to compensate for the failure of the thyroid to supply enough energy.

In this context, one particular factor, in contradiction to the generally received ideas, was to cause the incipient cancer process to accelerate—Carol's vegetarian diet. The prime mover was a drastic reduction in protein consumption and particularly in directly assimilated proteins, i.e. animal proteins, obliging the organism to increase its own production of proteins in order to supply the cell nuclei. When Carol compensated for this lack of protein with an increased consumption of dairy products, there were two disastrous consequences:

- An increase in the inflammatory process, and hence in the stimulation of immunoglobulins and a perverse acceleration of the tryptic: pancreas, adrenals and thyroid;
- An amplification of compensatory glucidic and lipidic activity and, again, over stimulation of the whole pancreas with an obligatory increase in the work of the liver.

This carcinogenic-type adaptation took two years to set in place, coinciding with the end of the second year of restructuring—that is, when Carol was 44. When in 1996 it was suggested that she start hormone replacement therapy, she was in the middle of the final year of restructuring—which is always the most dangerous.

Taking these hormones suddenly increased her folliculinic stimulation a hundred fold, particularly all the compensatory phenomena and the manufacturing process that these involve —notably the thyreotropic activity with its metabolic consequences, which are both direct (mainly in the liver) and indirect (general metabolic effects on the bones). All this helped to increase the cancerous process in these secondary zones, which proves that this is a general process, not one caused by metastatic cells. The process again accelerated when the original tumor was removed—an intervention that necessarily stimulates cellular and tissular growth to ensure healing.

The stress of romantic engagement and marriage at first would have increased the phenomena of aromatization as a result of the change in the rhythm and way of life that living with somebody else involves. Happily, love is a wonderful stimulant of one's survival instinct and of one's desire to live and hence of all the mechanisms of immune protection.

A Summary of Carol's Consultations with Dr. Lapraz

Following is a summary of Carol's visits with Dr. Lapraz as well as an explanation of the medicines that were prescribed to bring her body into balance. To facilitate the reading of the consultations, it is important to understand a few basic facts about the endocrine system:

- It is the body's management and information system.
- It works independently, without any conscious intervention on our part.
- It is organized on an hierarchical basis with control centers at the hypothalamus and pituitary levels. These control centers manage glands through two types of hormones: stimulating and inhibiting.
- Secretions of the endocrine glands (adrenal, ovary, thyroid, etc.) are carried to their final destination through the blood and are managed by the control centers through a feedback system.
- Organs and tissues receptors are the receivers of the hormones secretions, and initiate the requested metabolic effects.

- There are four hormonal axes: corticotrope, gonadotrope, thyreotrope and somatotrope. They function vertically (control centers to glands to receptors, specific to the axis) and horizontally, sometimes interfering with each other.

- The corticotrope axis manages the reaction of the body to an aggression (called the "adaptation syndrome"). This is a series of physiological actions aimed at driving the body's response to an aggression.

- The gonadotrope axis is a provider of raw materials and ensures protein synthesis, which contributes at the cellular level to growth, muscle development and bone reconstruction.

- The thyreotrope axis activates energy supplies by increasing the metabolism, and acts on the somatotrope axis to initiate building efforts at the cellular level.

- The somatotrope axis does the building work. It is comprised of growth factors (i.e., growth hormone GH) and anti-growth factors (i.e., somatostatin hormone), resulting in net growth that corresponds to normal cellular renewal in a healthy body.

- In the case of cancer, with the uncontrolled growth of malignant cells, it is vital to follow the relative functioning of these four axis very closely, because their interdependency plays a crucial role in the development of the disease and the patient's ability to overcome its troubles and establish a new balance.

- Endobiogénie's unique diagnostic tool, the Biology of Functions, tracks a large number of indexes which indicate factors favoring uncontrolled cell development. The summary indexes differentiate between the concept of a carcinogenic structure, which indicates elements potentially favoring uncontrolled cell development (i.e., at risk level), and the effective deployment of that risk, illustrated by the enlargement of existing tumors or the emergence of new ones.

February 2001: Carol's first visit occurred three years after the identification of a left breast cancer in December 1997, followed by a liver metastasis in November 1999, and a small metastatic tumor on the last left rib in February 2000. The cancer had followed a 16 month long estro-progestative hormone therapy when she was pre-menopausal in 1996. A CT scan was made a week before this visit, and it showed a new lesion in her liver. Carol's tumor marker CA15-3 was at 69.5 (normal range being 0-31.3).

The initial Biology of Functions provided the following information regarding the endocrine axes:

- Corticotrope axis: the secretion activity of the adrenal cortex was very high in response to a strong inflammation. The low level of the stimulating hormone ACTH (from the pituitary) shows that the activity of ACTH is exclusively directed towards maintaining a high glucocorticoid activity—therefore, the threshold of response of cortisol is very high, and there is insufficient ACTH for the rest of its endocrine and metabolic activities. The prolactin index was also very high, indicating an over stimulation of the production of androgens and estrogens. The histamine index was very high, indicating congestion in the areas of hyper-estrogenic activity, particularly in the liver.

- Gonadotrope axis: strong estrogenic activity (3 to 4 times the norm) and hyper folliculinic activity increasing the number of estrogen receptors and stimulating the development of the cancer.

- Thyreotrope axis: the metabolic activity of the thyroid was relatively low, which was a positive factor, since it protects the nucleus of the cell (which contains the DNA) by increasing insulin resistance. This was an important factor in Carol's case because the thyroid itself was very much implicated in her illness process (five times the norm).

- Carcinogenic assessment: most indexes were in the red area, such as adenosis (hyperplasia), fibrosis (congestion), growth factors, (stimulants of cancerous development), cell and DNA fractures. Some indexes however were positive, such as a strong apoptosic activity (the programmed death of cells which is usually reduced when cancer is developing), and high anti-growth factors (which slow the development of the tumor, in contrast to growth factors which stimulate it) indicating the potential of the organism to combat the illness over the long term.

- Metabolic activity: the turnover index was very high (four times the norm), indicating a slowdown in cell renewal, which is always consistent with a strong cancerous development. The pro-amyloid index was very high, indicating respiratory and nutritional insufficiencies at cell level. Bone remodeling was very high (four times the norm), indicating further risks of bone metastasis.

In summary, Carol's endobiogénie was very unstable, although her organism showed a raised defensive potential, as highlighted above. The objective of the treatment was to reduce the estrogenic activity and slow the three hormonal axes: gonadotrope (FSH, for the production of estrogens), thyreotrope (TSH, for the distribution of energy) and somatotrope (GH, for growth factors that encourage cancerous development). It was also important to reduce her pelvic congestion and rebalance her autonomic nervous system (and particularly to reduce alphasympathetic activity).

The main lines of the treatment and the medicinal plants used after this first consultation were as follows:

- In order to slow down the gonadotrope axis: *Lithospermum officinale* (gromwell).
- To block the estrogen receptors in order to balance androgenic activity: *Sequoia gigantea*, which also encourages bone reconstruction after the bone metastasis of February 2000.

- To correct the corticotrope axis: *Ribes nigrum* (blackcurrant), which stimulates the adrenal glands.

- To slow down prolactin and growth hormone: *Poterium sanguisorba* (great burnet).

- To slow down the thyroid axis and the transformation of T4 into T3 (the two thyroid hormones, which play a role in increasing energy): *Lycopus europaeus* (gypsywort), *Fabiana imbricata* (pichi).

- To reduce the pelvic congestion through venous stimulation: *Quercus spiritus glandulosus* (oak).

- To rebalance the autonomic nervous system by slowing down the alphasympathetic: *Vitex agnus castus* (chasteberry).

- To assure the correct functioning of the digestive system and drain the liver: *Chrysanthellum americanum, Chelidonium majus* (greater celandine), *Tilia europaea* (sapwood of lime).

- To sustain the immune system: *Viscum album querci* (oak mistletoe).

- To lift energy levels and revitalize the body: vitamin C and magnesium.

Two other recommendations were to stop the progesterone medication being taken (Megace) and to adapt nutrition to the cancer environment by eliminating dairy, wheat and soy from Carol's diet. The first two tend to cause inflammation and create allergies by stimulating the production of immunoglobulins, and soy contains estrogens. She was also encouraged to restart chemotherapy if her oncologist would agree to it.

May 2001: Two months before, Carol had restarted chemotherapy in tablet form using Xeloda. Its side effects were more bearable (no hair loss), but there was some diarrhea, and irritation on the palms of the hands and soles of the feet. There were signs of an improvement in her general state. The tumor marker CA15-3 was reduced by 9 points to 60.9, the estrogens reduced by 25%, the carcinogenic index reduced from 173 to 18, the thyroid involvement index reduced by 40%, and the anti-growth factors were becoming stronger, with the somatostatin index moving from 6 to 25. The resistance to the aggression was starting to become organized.

November 2001: The physiological endobiogenic data showed continuing improvement: Carol's tumor markers were in the normal range for the first time (30.99), turnover was down 70% (which means cell renewal is reactivated), estrogens down 30%, carcinogenic indexes down 70%, histamine down 60%, and growth factors close to normal. But a new stress had started to affect her organism, a stress coming from her business life, exacerbated by the events of 9/11: the adrenocortical index jumped to over four times the norm and its stimulating hormone, ACTH, jumped from 12 to 472 against a norm of 0.7 to 3. The DHEA index jumped from 24 to 3248 (DHEA is an androgen produced by the adrenal glands, which can be transformed into estrogens), against a norm of 5 to 9. All facts pointed to a possible reactivation of the pathology. The main lines of the treatment were maintained and reinforced by adding *Fragaria vesca* (strawberry root), to slow down the ACTH and inhibit the transformation of androgens into estrogens.

May 2002: Carol had made a decision to sell her company, which was the primary reason for her stress. However, this process was stressful in itself and it was to take her another year to extricate herself completely. The tumor marker continued to improve within the normal range at 24. The adrenocortical index, as well as the DHEA index (down to 78), had dropped very significantly, but there were signs that the pathology had regained momentum. Turnover was up again (indicating a drop in cellular renewal) and so were the estrogens, sustained by a jump in prolactin. The carcinogenic indexes were up, and so were the growth factors and the histamine.

October 2002: Carol had completed the sale of her business during the summer, making sure that all of her employees and suppliers had been properly provided for. But success always comes with a cost. Carol's stress jumped again, but not as much as in November 01: the adrenocortical index had increased eightfold and the DHEA had almost doubled to 153.

The effects of the previous stress on the pathology were devastating. The carcinogenic indexes were near the level they were at eighteen months before. The growth factors and adenosis were at a record high. The tumor marker however continued to improve within the norms at 20.5. (This shows the limits of a tumor marker measurement, which gives the level of a protein circulating in the blood. It correctly reflects the present or past situation, but not endobiogenic disturbances, which precede the reactivation of an illness, as the biology of functions indexes show.)

The main lines of the treatment were maintained and reinforced with seven new medications aimed at revitalizing the organism, reducing congestion, and supporting the eliminatory functions (liver, kidney,...).

Carol's thyroid was finally functioning properly and she was given a prescription for a number of fruit diets aimed at improving elimination, and also to help her lose weight:

- A lemon juice regime for 21 days to increase the fluidity of the blood and to reduce the risk of circulatory problems (this was to be taken in addition to her regular diet). She had to boil a lemon and then extract the juice, starting with one lemon the first day, two the next and so on up to ten lemons, and then reverse this routine (10, 9, 8...). This lemon juice regime was to be followed every other month starting in November.

- A melon diet, for its diuretic effect, starting with a three-day lead-in period (brown rice only on the first day, vegetables only on the second and fruit only on the third day), then four days of melons only and then the same in reverse sequence. Again, this diet was to be done for ten days only every other month, starting in November.

- A pineapple diet, which is basically the same as the melon diet, but instead of four days of melons only, it consists of brown rice, olive oil and pineapple (with the same lead-in, etc. as the melon diet), for its action in reducing fat levels. This was to alternate month by month with the melon diet, which meant that it would start in December.

May 2003: The stress was now history and, for the first time, nearly everything was going in the right direction:

- Adrenal activity down, with the DHEA at 26 versus 153 in October 02.
- Turnover down to 82, its lowest level for the past two years (norm is 40 to 60), indicating an increase in cellular renewal.
- Carcinogenic indices down significantly from last October's peak.
- Adenosis (hyperplasia factor) down to 42 from 6105 last October (norm 10 to 30).
- Growth factors within the norms, down 80% from last October.
- Estrogens still high but much better balanced with the androgens.
- Histamine however had gone up and was at twice the norm, feeding the congestion.
- Weight had come down five-and-a-half pounds.
- The tumor marker (CA 15-3) remained stable at 23.3.

October 2003: Carol's health parameters had improved very significantly. The positive directions of last May were confirmed across the board, and many indexes were back to normal:

- Adrenal activity within norms: DHEA down 26 to 4.3 (within norms).
- Estrogens down (20% since May), still above the norms, but well balanced with androgens.

- Progesterone down (25%) and within norms.
- Turnover down (30% since May) and within norms.
- Carcinogenic indexes down very significantly, nearly within norms.
- Adenosis down from 42 to 2.6 (norm 10 to 30).
- Growth factors down further and within norms.
- Histamine down 127 to 78 (norms 20 to 60).
- Pro-amyloid index back within the norms, indicating a regular flow of energy at cell level.
- Bony remodeling down 70% over the past 2 years and close to the norms.
- Metabolic activity (catabolism and anabolism) remaining high as well as contribution of the thyroid involvement to the pathology.
- Weight down almost another 9 pounds. She had lost about 15 pounds over the last 12 months.

May 2004: Physiological parameters were well stabilized. A few more improvements:

- Corticotropic axis normalized. DHEA down to 1.8.
- Estrogens normalized for the first time: estrogens down to 0.37 from 0.62 in October.
- Androgenic index down from 0.48 to 0.27 and within norms.
- Progesterone stabilized within norms.
- Growth and anti-growth factors within norms.
- Histamine (driver of congestion) stable as well as carcinogenic indices.
- Metabolic activity back within the norms.
- Weight down a further nine pounds, reaching her normal weight of 123 pounds.

December 2004: Carol's state had deteriorated as a result of a number of repetitive stresses, and a CT scan, on December 10, highlighted two new tumors in her liver. The CA 15-3 tumor marker did not yet reflect this deterioration, although it had slightly increased to 24.2 (norm less or equal to 30).

This deterioration can also be attributed to an increase in thyroid activity towards the end of menopause, which usually does not generate any particular problem in the absence of pathology. This burst of thyroid activity is associated with a sharp increase in metabolism, very visible on Carol's Biology of Functions (metabolic yield moving from 57 in May to 270 in December, against a norm of 80 to 140) and with an equally sharp increase in androgens and estrogens, which increased by between 40% and 90%.

In the case of Carol, this burst of thyroid activity changed the local intrahepatic metabolism in specific areas, because receptors to thyroid hormones are more concentrated in specific parts of the liver. This explains why two pre-existing tumors, microscopic in size, had grown to the point where they had become visible while other liver tumors remained stable. This kind of situation could reoccur in the future, but this does not alter the fact that her organism overall was moving towards a new balance of coexistence with her pathology.

Certain aspects of Carol's treatment were reinforced in order to reduce thyroid activity (*Fabiana imbricata, Lycopus europaeus*) and genital hormone activity (*Lithospermum officinale*), and to strengthen the adrenal cortex (*Ribes nigrum*) in order to better manage stress.

May 2005: Carol's state normalized at the best level she had achieved since February 2001. She had achieved a level of internal balance, reflecting full control of her body, including the metastases. She was in a situation similar to that of pregnancy, as indicated by her pregnancy index, which increased to 5.5 against a norm of between 1 to 2. One should recall that, during pregnancy, the organism reacts first in a attitude of mistrust, as it does during the installation of a new tumor (sharp increase of fibrosis in particular), then accepts the pregnancy and integrates it in its hormonal activities. The pregnancy index measures the acceptance and the tolerance of a foreign body developing within the organism and recognized for what it is. Carol's index jumped from 0.4 in March to 5.5 in May, indicating a high level of acceptance of her metastases by her organism.

Carol's last CT scan shows stability in the size of the tumors, and the CA 15-3 marker, which tends to react with a time lag, remains above the norm at 51.

The main features revealed by the clinical exam were an over-activity of the thyroid and an excessive adaptational activity, which is demonstrated in particular by:

- A pulse of over 90, whatever the circumstances.
- Signs of TSH activity below the left clavicle and left axilla, under the left ankle and in the outer upper quadrant of the left breast.
- A light TSH activity just below the inside knee.
- An LH reactivity maintaining the TSH activity (shown by signs more evident in the left breast than the right), probably because of the necessary role thyroid hormones play in a mechanism, already installed, which uses uterine estrogen receptors.
- A strong increase in insulin, which acts in anticipation of efforts at adaptation and in compensation for the delayed increase in GH and the decrease in estrogens that is characteristic of the end of menopause.

Carol's treatment was continued overall in order to reduce thyroid, genital and GH activity, while strengthening the immune system and supporting the pancreas and the liver.

August 2005: The June CT scan revealed the increase of three tumors in Carol's liver, without new lesions. At the same time, the CA 15-3 continued the steady growth initiated in March, moving from 44 to 71. Treatment with Xeloda was maintained at the same frequency that Dr. Woliver had switched her to in December (two weeks on, one week off).

The August 26 Biology of Functions shows a sharp deterioration versus May, amplified by stress linked with the death of Carol's mother-in-law:

- Corticotrope axis up on the front line, an indication of a strong response to the new aggression: cortisol up 4 times from a normal level (6.3 to 26.7), same for adrenal gland activity doubled (3.2 to 6.9), serotonin and peripheral aldosterone, which play key roles in support of the adaptation, considerably increased from normal levels, up respectively by factors 8 and 300. As a consequence, the adrenal gland reduced its permissive role by 50% towards other hormonal axis. Inflammation is up five times (1 to 5.1) from a normal level

- Gonadotrope axis is activated on the metabolic front through genital hormones, while tissular estrogenic activities are increasing, particularly in periphery.

- Thyreotrope axis still normal at both thyroid and upstream levels

- Somatotrope axis deteriorating: GH activity increased 50% from a normal level (5.5 to 11.2), anti-growth activity reduced 40%, insulin increased 60% but within norm, insulin resistance sharply reduced from a normal level (0.9 to 0.09), while oxydoreduction is increased 90 times from a low level (0.2 to 18.5), and apoptosis is reduced by near 80% from a normal level

- All factors which reactivate the cancer more at structure level (up 14 times) than in its effective deployment. Adenosis, however, an indicator of hyperplasia activity, is up 3 times.

The treatment was reinforced twice for reducing genital hormone metabolic activities: by increasing the the dose of *Vitex agnus castus*

(Chasteberry) and by adding *Borago* (Borage). The dose of *Lycopus europaea* (Bugleweed) and *Brassica oleracea* (Cabbage) was increased 2.5 times to further control the upstream level of the thyreotrope axis, while a number of tools were maintained to inhibit cancer cells proliferation: injections of *Viscum Quercus* (Oak mistletoe), *Chelidonium* (Celandine), anti-oxydants

January 2006: The most recent CT scan shows that three lesions are further enlaged, but that there are no new ones:

- CA 15-3 continues regular growth: 71 in August, 104 in November, and 160 in January.
- A decision is made to stop Xeloda chemotherapy and switch to Doxil, which is started on January 23

The January Biology of Functions is at its worst levels for several years:

- Corticotrope axis hyperactive: cortisol at peak (33.1), adrenal gland (5.4) strong enough however to support the high level of adaptation
- Gonadotrope axis deteriorating: metabolic activities increased 50% (both androgens and estrogens), tissular activities increased 70 to 100%
- Thyreotrope axis remains normal at both thyroid and upstream levels
- Somatotrope axis hyper active: growth hormone activity up, anti-growth reduced, overall growth score increased five times, cells renewal reduced, apostosis further reduced.
- As a result, the carcinogenic structure increases substantially vs August (+60%) and its effective deployment continues to deteriorate (up 3 times). Adenosis is equally up 20% vs August.

The escape of the disease, in spite of chemotherapy and endobiogenic treatment, should be considered in the context of the multiple stresses which affect life, particularly during a long-standing disease such as Carol's. Such situations do occur and they are recoverable, if the mental outlook of the patient is strong enough. Carol will prove once more that she could overcome this challenge.

Treatment changes: increase immune function (injections of *Viscum album*), stimulate adrenal function and reduce alphasympathetic (*Gentiana* with *Thymus* and *Melissa*), protect liver functions (*Curcuma* with *Boldo* and *Combretum*), increase dose of anti-gonadotrope plants (*Lithospermum officinale* and *Poterium Sanguisorba*).

March 2006: The most recent CT scan shows further deterioration with multiple new lesions:

- CA 15-3 continues to deteriorate: 160 in January, 225 in February, 276 in March

- Decision to stop Doxil and to move back to Xeloda, combined with Gemzar

The March Biology of Functions worsens on the thyreotrope axis, which has immediate implications for aggravating the disease, although the other axes tend to improve:

- Corticotrope axis: adaptation down (cortisol reduced 33.1 to 13.3, adrenal gland reduced 5.4 to 2.1)

- Gonadotrope axis: gonads metabolic and tissular activities reduce 30–50%

- Thyreotrope axis: strong reactivation at both thyroid and upstream levels. The thyroidal implication in the disease is nearly doubled, and the upstream hormone (TRH) is doubling its activity with the pancreas, which reactivates insulin and reduces insulin resistance, hence contributing to the proliferation of new lesions.

- Somatotrope axis: growth hormone activity reduced while anti-growth is up, reducing considerably the overall growth score. Oxydo reduction, however, is strongly increased, which contributes to the growth of the lesions

- The carcinogenic structure however, in terms of risk parameters, improves from its January peak, but the strength of the TRH remains a major exposure

Treatment changes: reinforcement of the thyreotrope axis (*Lycopus europa* and *Brassica oleracea*)

August 2006: a CT scan at the end of April showed further progression of the disease, with new lesions in both lobes of the liver:

- Gemzar is stopped in May and replaced by Faslodex in combination with Xeloda
- CA 15-3 continues to deteriorate: 276 in March, 435 in June, and 1020 in August
- Decision made in July to put a final stop to Xeloda. It is replaced by Methotrexate and Cytoxan, with Aromasin added early August and Triptorelin late August

The August Biology of Functions shows a continued worsening of the situation versus March:

- Corticotrope axis: adaptation level substantially increased to fight the worsening of the disease (cortisol up again 13.3 to 35.2, adrenal gland activity up 2.1 to 8.8 at 2.5 times the norm). Inflammation at a peak up 4 times vs March
- Gonadotrope axis: stable at March level on metabolic activities and increasing on tissular activities
- Thyreotrope axis deteriorating sharply, driven by a strong beta sympathetic stimulating the upstream hormone (TRH) reaching a peak on its impact over pancreas
- Somatotrope axis deteriorating vs March with growth hormone activity up, anti-growth down and, in consequence, the net growth score up six times. This contributes to a sharp increase of the carcinogenesis structure, although not to the level of January 06.

Treatment changes: reduce inflammation (Inflamease), reduce thyreotrope axis activity (*Brassica oleracea*, *Brassica napus* and *Fabiana imbricata*), reduce insulin activity (*Malva sylvestris* and *Arnica*), protect and drain liver (*Carduus marianus, Chrysantellum americanum*), reduce oxydation activity (CoQ10)

December 2006: A CT scan in November shows a turnaround for the first time with a diminution of the extensive metastatic disease in the liver:

- CA 15-3 shows the same turnaround after the peak reached in September: 1020 in August, 1440 in September, 1280 in October, 1080 in November, and 614 in December

- Decision to stop hormonal therapy in September and start on a new chemotherapy (Abraxane) September 13.

The December Biology of Functions shows a mixed picture vs August, three months after the change in chemotherapy:

- Corticotrope axis: adaptation remains strong (cortisol up 35 to 41, six times the norm) but it is well managed by the adrenal gland, which is active enough to handle both adaptation and its permissive role towards other hormonal axis.

- Gonadotrope axis further improved in both metabolic and tissular activities, the latter however remaining high, with estrogens predominant over androgens to support the bone tissular activity (see below)

- Thyreotrope axis significantly improved throughout metabolic and tissular activities, with a TRH upstream also improved in its relationship with pancreas (reduced 20%) which helps reducing insulin by nearly 80%, while increasing insulin resistance by a factor 10.

- Somatotrope axis perturbed by a temporary hyper anabolism in the bones (bone isoenzymes at twice the norm in November/December) which increases the growth hormone activity and the anti-growth factors, resulting in a jump of the net growth score at 7 times the norm. The pancreas activity however is reduced as indicated above (drop of insulin and increased insulin resistance), which slows down cancer cells activity. One last point to mention: a very large conges-tion of the liver (activity increased over 100 times), a consequence of multiple change in medications throughout 2006: this congestion will disappear in 2 months, after a Melissa treatment

- As a result of the growth hyperactivity in the bones area, the carcino-genic structure deteriorates sharply by a factor 20, indicating a higher risk for the proliferation of the disease, but the effective deployment of this risk reduces, in line with the trend of the CA 15/3

Treatment changes: further reduce thyreotrope axis activity (*Zea mais*), drain liver (*Pneumus Boldo, Cichorium*), eliminate liver congestion (*Combretum* and *Melissa*), regulate oxydation and protect from vascular risks (*Gingko*)

March 2007: a CT scan on February 8 shows that the tumors continue to reduce in size:

- CA 15-3 is slightly up since December: 614 in December, 638 in January, 716 in February
- Avastin is added to Abraxane on March 20

The March Biology of Functions shows improvements vs December 2006, with one exception—the adaptation effort remains high, but it will abate over the following months:

- Corticotrope axis: adaptation increased 41 to 71, versus December 06. The adrenal gland activity is reduced substantially, which prevents playing an effective role versus other hormonal axis
- Gonadotrope axis: stability of the metabolic contribution and sub-stantial reduction of tissular activities, with a rebalance estrogens/androgens in favor of androgens
- Thyreotrope axis: thyroid within norm across metabolic and tissular activities. The TRH is in slight increase driven this time by the thyroid reduction downstream.

- Somatotrope axis: GH activity is down near norm, while anti-growth activity is also down within norm. The insulin activity is stable within norm, while insulin resistance is down from a high level in February, with no adverse effect

- The carcinogenic structure is sharply down, as well as its effective deployment

Treatment changes: reinforce anti inflammatory function (*Plantago major*), slow down androgens metabolic and tissular activities (*Serenoa, Pygeum africanum*)

August 07: A CT scan on June 7 shows continued reduction in the size of the liver lesions:

- CA 15/-3 has some ups and downs but the trend is going down: 716 in March, 645 in May, 490 in June, 445 in August.

The August Biology of Functions is one of the very best of the past three years. Nearly all indicators are green with one exception: the reactivation of TRH to its March level, after a drop in June, in its relationship with the pancreas, which generates a rebound of the insulin activity. But this time it did not generate a decrease in insulin resistance, because of a strengthening somatostatin (see below) :

- Corticotrope axis: adaptation near norm (down 71 to 12), adrenal gland normal and activity towards other hormonal axis increased towards norm

- Gonadotrope axis: metabolic activities down to norm, tissular activities down to norm for estrogens and still high for androgens, while estrogens tissular activity is down in periphery

- Thyreotrope axis: normalized (metabolism, yield, tissular activity) with one exception, the rebound of the TRH mentioned above

- Somatotrope axis: significant improvement with a number of indicators back to norm: growth hormone activity down 50% to norm, anti-growth adjusted downward within norm, insulin however doubled (1.7 to 4.0) but without adverse effect on insulin resistance, which is strengthened by the growth of the somatostatin (growth hormone inhibitor) more than doubled. Overall net growth score is normalized, as well as metabolism and cells renewal, there is no congestion, and adenosis is sharply down

- Carcinogenesis: best record over the past 3 years with structure and deployment down significantly and within norms

Treatment is maintained with reinforced liver protection (*Curcuma*).

In Summary

Carol's health is as good as she could have hoped, and it's been eight years since the cancer in her breast metastasized to her liver. At that time she was given two years to live and a three-percent chance of conquering the disease.

How can we understand such an evolution of the pathology that is so different from the one expected eight years ago? We believe that the endobiogenic treatment has properly taken into account the various physiological mechanisms, which ensure the overall balance of Carol's organism. The tracking of these physiological mechanisms through the Biology of Functions model has been the constant reference for the selection of the endobiogenic therapeutic elements, in harmony with her hormonal and chemotherapy treatment, in order to help Carol's organism to achieve a better state of equilibrium, by removing those dysfunctions that are feeding the development of her cancer.

The combination of chemotherapy, when necessary, with endobiogenic treatment, supports and adjusts the equilibrium of the organism, and offers a major opportunity for cancer patients. Anyone suffering from cancer should be able to enjoy the considerable benefits provided by an endobiogenic approach.

Carol's personal involvement in her treatment has been an important factor in its success. She has taken many aspects of her life under control, and made necessary changes in her professional life, nutrition, and activities. She has learned to adapt to her disease by thinking of cancer as a chronic illness, rather than considering it a failure that she could not be immediately and completely cured. This has helped her remain vigilant and continue the endobiogenic treatment on a daily basis—which keeps her body in balance.

Graphs Illustrating Carol's Biology of Functions

To illustrate the complexity of Carol's treatment, we have attached a few graphs (from among hundreds) that clearly show how the Biology of Functions allows one to closely follow the evolution of the disease. By using this tool, the practitioner can identify changes in the patient's equilibrium—even when no clinical signs are present—and can adjust the treatment in order to prevent a resurgence of the disease.

Carol's Levels of the Breast Cancer Tumor Marker CA 15-3

NORMAL RANGE IS 30 OR LESS

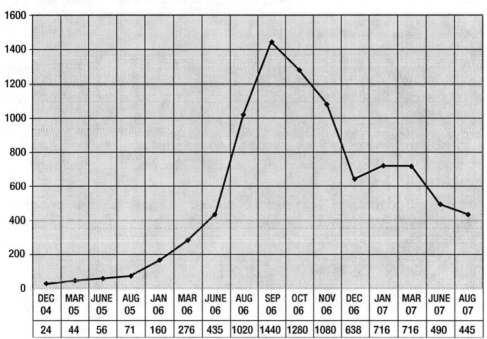

DEC 04	MAR 05	JUNE 05	AUG 05	JAN 06	MAR 06	JUNE 06	AUG 06	SEP 06	OCT 06	NOV 06	DEC 06	JAN 07	MAR 07	JUNE 07	AUG 07
24	44	56	71	160	276	435	1020	1440	1280	1080	638	716	716	490	445

The evolution of CA 15-3 shows a continuous deterioration from March 2005, which is when Carol's organism started escaping Xeloda. Alternative chemotherapy and hormonal therapy was applied until finally being replaced by Abraxane in September 2006, when the CA 15-3's rising trend started to abate.

Carol's Estrogenic Metabolic Activity
NORMAL RANGE IS 0.20 TO 0.40

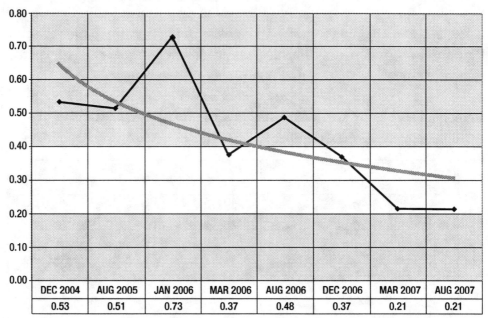

	DEC 2004	AUG 2005	JAN 2006	MAR 2006	AUG 2006	DEC 2006	MAR 2007	AUG 2007
	0.53	0.51	0.73	0.37	0.48	0.37	0.21	0.21

The graph and the one on the facing page illustrate Carol's estrogenic and androgenic metabolic activities. They have a similar pattern to the CA 15-3 graph, which reached a peak in January 2006.

Carol's Androgenic Metabolic Activity
NORMAL RANGE IS 0.20 TO 0.25

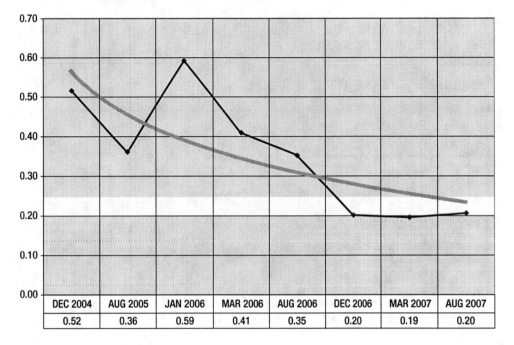

DEC 2004	AUG 2005	JAN 2006	MAR 2006	AUG 2006	DEC 2006	MAR 2007	AUG 2007
0.52	0.36	0.59	0.41	0.35	0.20	0.19	0.20

Carol's Thyroid Yield
NORMAL RANGE IS 2.00 TO 3.00

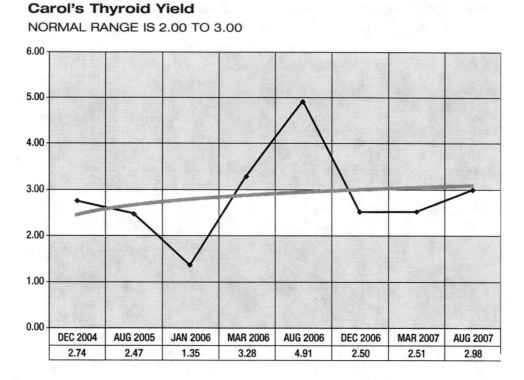

DEC 2004	AUG 2005	JAN 2006	MAR 2006	AUG 2006	DEC 2006	MAR 2007	AUG 2007
2.74	2.47	1.35	3.28	4.91	2.50	2.51	2.98

The thyroid yield graph has a different pattern. The peak was reached in August 2006, driven by a strong TRH upstream, which was stimulated by a strong beta-sympathetic reaction. It is about the same time that the CA 15-3 hits its peak.

Carol's DNA Fracture
NORMAL RANGE IS 2.00 TO 3.00

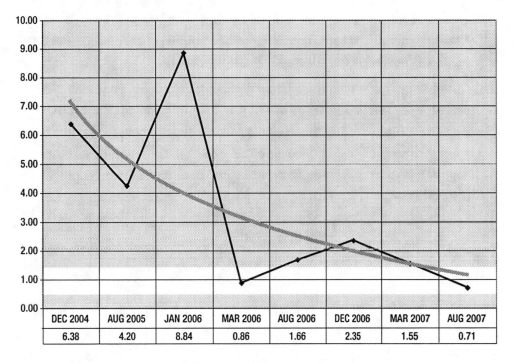

	DEC 2004	AUG 2005	JAN 2006	MAR 2006	AUG 2006	DEC 2006	MAR 2007	AUG 2007
	6.38	4.20	8.84	0.86	1.66	2.35	1.55	0.71

Carol's DNA Fracture hit its peak in January 2006, as did the estrogens and metabolic activities. This was the signal for the new tumor activities that lasted until September 2006.

A closing note from Carol Silverander:

> *This concludes the section written by Drs. Lapraz and Duraffourd. Hopefully it will give readers a better understanding of endobiogénie and the role it has played in the treatment of my cancer.*

> *I truly hope this book will help many patients refuse the prognosis of a programmed death and let go of the fear and, in so doing, learn to live with their disease rather than being overcome by it. I know that stabilizing my cancer will be an ongoing battle and that there will be ups and downs. Life itself is not stagnant, but flows like a river. I am prepared for the challenge.*

BIBLIOGRAPHY

Acupuncture.com/newsletters, **"Acupuncture for Cancer—Integrating Eastern with Western Medicine,"** Fay-Meling von Moltke Pao, DAc, BHSc, Hon.BA, http://www.acupuncture.com/newsletters/m_dec05/main2.htm

American Dental Association, **"Osteoneucrosis of the Jaw,"** www.ada.org/prof/resources/topics/osteonecrosis.asp

Annals of Oncology, **"Faslodex Benefits Subset of Women Resistant to Aromatase Inhibitors,"** Perey L, Paridaens, R, Hawle H et al. 2007;18:64-69. Final results of Phase II Swiss Group for Clinical Cancer Research Trial (SAKK 21/00).

Annals of Oncology, **"Low-dose methotrexate and cyclophosphamide in metastatic breast cancer: antitumor activity and correlation with vascular endothelial growth factor levels,"** M. Colleoni, A. Rocca, M.T. Sandri, L. Zorzino, G. Masci, F. Nolè, G. Peruzzotti, C. Robertson, L. Orlando, S. Cinieri, F. de Braud, G. Viale and A. Goldhirsch. Received 29 March 2001,; revised 26 June 2001; accepted 5 July 2001. Volume 13, Number 1> Pp. 73-80.

Associated Press, **"Cancer Research Fails to Meet Doctors' Expectations,"** Daniel Q. Haney, July 28, 2003. (Contra Costa Times) www.bayarea.com

Associated Press, **"Hormone Linked to Breast Cancer."** Lindsey Tanner, Chicago, September 13, 2002. (Detroit News) www.detnews.com

Associated Press, **"New Drug Better for Preventing Breast Tumors, Arimidex Benefits Women with Early-Stage Breast Cancer."** (MSNBC) www.msnbc.com

Associated Press, **"New Drug Delays Breast Cancer (Tykerb),"** June 3, 2006. Atlanta, www.wired.com

BBC News, **"New Pill Helps Breast Cancer Care."** March 15, 2004 http://news.bbc.co.uk

BBC News, **"Twins Clue to Breast Cancer."** July 23, 2002. http://news.bbc.co.uk

The Boston globe (boston.com), Health sense, **"Women Continue to Demand Hormones Despite Research."** Judy Foreman, Globe Staff, March 9, 2004. www.boston.com

Breastcancer.org, **"Abraxane Better than Taxol for Advanced Breast Cancer."** http://www.breastcancer.org/research_recurrence_022405.html

Breastcancer.org, **"Avastin Given with Taxol Slows Advanced Breast Cancer."** K. D. Miller et al. San Antonio Breast Cancer Symposium, December 8, 2005, Abstract 3. http://www.breastcancer.org/research_recurrence_021706.html

Breastcancer.org, **"Doxil, A new Type of Adriamycin, has Fewer Serious Side Effects."** M.O'Brien et al. Annals of Oncology Volume 15, March 2004. http://www.breastcancer.org/research_chemotherapy_doxil.html

Breastcancer.org, **"Feb. 2005: Updates from St. Gallen."** Primary Therapy of Early Breast Cancer Conference, St. Gallen, Switzerland, January 2005, Abstract #S4. http://www.breastcancer.org

Breastcancer.org, **"Fewer Side Effects with Sentinel Lymph Node Removal."** San Antonio Breast Cancer Symposium, December 2004, Abstracts #15,18. http://www.breastcancer.org

The Canadian Women's Health Network, **"HRT in the news The Women's Health Initiative Study at a Glance."** Kathleen O'Grady, Director of Communications for the Canadian Women's Health Network and Editor of A Friend Indeed Newsletter, Sept/Oct. 2002. Also **"WHI, Estrogen and Progestin Trial,"** update (March 2004) www.cwhn.ca/resources/menopause/hrt-glance.html

CancerConsultants.com, **"ixabepilone Effective in MNetastatic Breast Cancer That Doesn't Respond to Standard Chemotherapy."** Cancer News, CancerConsultants.com, July 9, 2007. www.cancerconsultants.com

CancerConsultants.com, **"Oncotype DX Meets Blue Cross and Blue Shield Technology Evaluation Criteria."** Cancer News, CancerConsultants.com, July 23, 2007. www.cancerconsultants.com

CancerConsultants.com, **"Tykerb May Be Effective in Brain Metastasis from Breast Cancer."** Cancer News, CancerConsultants.com, July 23, 2007. www.cancerconsultants.com

CBS News, **"HRT-Dementia Warning Issued."** Lauran Neergaard, Associated Press, Washington, February 10, 2004.www.cbsnews.com

Channelnewsasia.com, **"New Drug Breast Cancer Arimidex™ Cuts Risk of Relapse: Study."** December 11, 2004. www.channelnewsasia.com

Chlebowski RT et al: **"Influence of Estrogen Plus Progestin on Breast Cancer and Mammography in Healthy Postmenopausal Women."** JAMA, July 17, 2002 vol. 289 no. 24

Cousins, Norman, **"Anatomy of an Illness."** W.W. Norton & Company, Inc., 1979.

Cousins, Norman, **"Head First: The Biology of Hope and the Healing Power of the Human Spirit."** Penguin Books USA, Inc., 1989.

Detroit Free Press, **"Hormone Supplements Raise Another Red Flag for Women,"** by Lindsey Tanner, The Associated Press, February 23, 2005. www.freep.com

The Cincinnati Enquirer, **"Cancer Drug Offers Hope."** Tim Bonfield www.enquirer.com

CNN.Com health>diet & fitness. **"New Research Supports Health Benefits of Red Wine."** From Staff Reports, July 3, 2000. www.cnn.com

Forbes.com, **"Breast Cancer Therapy Shows New Promise."** (Herceptin) Steven Reinberg, Health Day Reporter, May 19, 2004. www.forbes.com

Forbes.com, **"Tamoxifen Still a Potent Breast Cancer Therapy."** Amanda Gardner, Health Day Reporter. May 2, 2004. www.forbes.com

Guardian Unlimited, **"Breast Cancer Drug Dilemma."** Sarah Boseley, Health Editor. December 8, 2004. www.guardian.co.uk

Gemzar.com

Imaginis.com, **"Lymph Nodes–Breast Health"** and **"Breast Cancer Treatment–Lymphedema."** September, 2004. www.imaginis.com/breasthealth

Itnews, **"Arimidex™ Allows More Women to Live Free of Breast Cancer than Tamoxifen."** PR Newswire, December 12, 2004. www.itnews.it/risorse/EuroNews

Komen Foundation News, **"British Study Supports U.S. Findings on Hormone Replacement Therapy Risks."** August 11, 2003. www.komen.org

The Lancet, **"Breast Cancer and Hormone Replacement Therapy in the Million Women Study."** Million Women Study Collaborators, August 9, 2003. www.thelancet.com

LA Times.com, **"Study Suggests Link Between Stress and Breast Cancer."** Dianne Partie Lange, October 13, 2003.

Medical News Today, **"Arimidex™ (Anastrozole) better than Tamoxifen in Preventing Breast Cancer Recurrence."** December 8, 2004. www.medicalnewstoday.com

MSNBC, **"A Better Breast Cancer Drug?"** www.msnbc.com

MSNBC, **"New Breast Cancer Treatment Option."** Reuters, May 19, 2003 www.msnbc.com

National Dairy Council, **"Statement re: Jane Plant's statements regarding diet and nutrition are inaccurate and potentially harmful."** February 16, 2001.

Natural Health Line, **"Iscador shows Significant Promise in Major New Scientific Study."** Peter Chowka, May 1, 2001. http://naturalhealthline.com

News Services, **"Breast Cancer Drug Could Cause Uterine Cancer, FDA Warns."** June 28, 2002, Star Tribune. www.startribune.com

The New York Times, **"Citing Risks, U.S. Will Halt Study of Drugs for Hormones."** Gina Kolata, July 9, 2002. www.nytimes.com

The New York Times, **"Hormone Use Found to Raise Dementia Risk."** Denise Grady, May 28, 2003. www.nytimes.com

The New York Times, **"New Study Links Hormones to Breast Cancer Risk."** Lawrence Altman, August 8, 2003. www.nytimes.com

The New York Times, **"Study Finds New Risks in Hormone Therapy."** Denise Grady, June 25, 2003. www.nytimes.com

NHLBI Women's Health Initiative, **"Finds From The WHI Postmenopausal Hormone Therapy Trials."** April, 2004. www.nhlbi.nih.gov/whi

The Orange County Register, **"Somer's Cancer Treatment Decision Draws Questions."** Lisa Liddane, May 16, 2001.

PSA Rising, **"Short Course of Tibetan Yoga Improves Sleep in Cancer Patients."** Carla Warneke and Alma Rodriguez from M.D. Anderson Cancer Center; and Rachel Fouladi, Ph.D. from Simon Fraser university, april 23, 2004. http://psa-rising.com

The Quotable Woman. Running Press, 1991.

Regulatory Affairs News, **"British Women Shows Increased Cancer Risks From HRT."** April 29, 2004. www.raps.org

Reuters, **"ASCO - Bristol Drug Delays Breast Cancer Progression (Ixabepilone)."** Ransdell Pierson, June 3, 2007. www.reuters.com

Reuters, **"U.S. FDA Strengthens Hormone Warnings for Women."** Maggie Fox, January 9, 2003. www.enn.com

Seattle Post-Intelligencer Reporter, **"Hormone Study Finds Link to Lobular Breast Cancer."** Carol Smith, December 4, 2002. http://seattlepi.nwsource.com

Shumaker SA etal: **"Estrogen Plus Progestin and the Incidence of Dementia and Mild Cognitive Impairment in Postmenopausal Women."** JAMA, May 28, 2003 vol. 289 no. 20

Stanford Report. **"Yoga Class Designed to Meet Cancer Patients' Needs."** Michelle L. Brandt, December 4, 2002.

USA Today, **"Breast Cancer Risk Reduced by Exercise."** Rita Rubin http://usatoday.printthis.clickability.com

USA Today, Health & Science, **"New Research Clarifies Red Wine's Benefits."** Kathleen Fackelmann, USA Today. December 19, 2001. www.usatoday.com

The Wall Street Journal, **"Aventis Drug Aids Survival Rate in Early Stage of Breast Cancer."** Ron Winslow and Julia Flynn, December 8, 2003.

The Wall Street Journal, Personal Journal, A Special Report Personal Health, **"Why Curing Your Cancer May Not Be the Best Idea."** Tara Parker-Pope, February 11, 2003.

Washington Post.com, **"Drug Combination Approved for Breast Cancer."** (Xeloda and Taxotere), Associated Press, September 11, 2001, Page A09.

Washington Post.com, **"Drug Switch Could Reduce Breast Cancer Recurrence."** Rob Stein, Washington Post Staff Writer, March 11, 2004. www.washingtonpost.com

Washington Post.com, **"FDA Offers Guidance on Hormone Therapy."** Marc Kaufman, Washington Post Staff Writer, September 10, 2003; Page A03. www.washingtonpost.com

Washington Post.com, **"Genetic Test Is Predictor of Breast Cancer Relapse."** Rob Stein, Washington Post Staff Writer, December 11, 2004: Page A01 www.washingtonpost.com

Washington Post.com, **"Hormone Use's Link to Cancer Risk Reinforced."** Rob Stein, Washington Post Staff Writer, August 8, 2003, Page A02. www.washingtonpost.com

"Women's Health Initiative," JAMA, July 17, 2002 vol 288 no. 3.

The World Link.com, **"Study: New Breast Cancer Drug Better Than Tamoxifen."** Linda A. Johnson, Associated Press Writer, March 11, 2004. www.theworldlink.com

Yeshiva University News, **"Einstein Researcher Investigates the Healing Benefits of Yoga for Breast Cancer Patients."** Karen Gardner, January 16, 2004. http://news.yu.edu

Medical Test References

PET Scan – Positron Emission Tomography
www.falange.demon.co.uk/explain-petscan.htm

MUGA Scan – Multi Gated Acquisition. Marquette General Health System www.mgh.org/education/health/muga.html

MUGA Scan – "The MUGA Scan's role in Monitoring Cancer Therapy." Dr. Rich, September 28, 2000.
http://heartdisease.about.com/library/blmuga.htm

Radiation Cancer Treatment (Radiotherapy) Imaginis
http://imaginis.com/breasthealth/radiobetreatment

Femara Letrozole Tablets, Novartis Oncology.
www.us.femara.com

MRI – "How MRI Works." Todd A. Gould, RT-® (MR) (ARRT). How Stuff Works. http://electronics.howstuffworks.com

Brain Cancer Oncology Channel. Health Communities.com. Physician developed and monitored. March 9, 2004.
www.oncologychannel.com/braincancer/diagnosis.shtmlMRI

Scanning Information produced by doctors. Medicine Net.com
www.medicinenet.com/MRIscan/article.htm

Bone Scan – Nuclear Medicine. Marquette General Health System.
www.mgh.org/nuclear/bone.html

Bone Scan – Cancer Research UK www.cancerhelp.org.uk

Ultrasound – Christiana Care Health System
www.christianacare.org

Resources

American Academy of Medical Acupuncture
4929 Wilshire Boulevard, Suite 428
Los Angeles, CA 90010
323-937-5514 | www.medicalacupuncture.org

American Dental Association
211 East Chicago Avenue
Chicago, IL 60611-2678
312-440-2500 | www.ada.org/prof/resources/topics/osteonecrosis.asp

American Cancer Society
1-800-ACS-2345 | www.cancer.org

American Society of Clinical Oncology
1900 Duke Street, Suite 200
Alexandria, VA 22314
703-299-0150 | www.asco.org www.PeopleLivingWithCancer.org

Annie Appleseed Project, The
7319 Serrano Terrace
Delray Beach, FL 33446-2215
www.annieappleseedproject.org
email: annieappleseedpr@aol.com

Associations des Usagers de la Phytothérapie (PHYTO 2000)
www.phyto2000.org

Biology of Functions website
www.endobiogenics.com

Breastcancer.org
111 Forrest Avenue 1R
Narberth, PA 19072
Marisa C. Weiss, M.D., President and Founder
www.breastcancer.org

Cancer Care, Inc.
275 Seventh Avenue
New York, NY 10001
800-813-HOPE
www.cancercare.org

CancerConsultants.com
Oncology Resource Center
411 6th Street
Ketchum, ID 83340
www.cancerconsultants.com

Circle of Hope, Inc.
P.O. Box 221461
Newhall, CA 91322
Phone: 661-254-5218
www.circleofhopeinc.org

Endobiogenic Integrative Medical Center (EIMC)
357 W. Center, Suite 204
Pocatello, ID 83204
Phone/Fax: 208-478-8400 | Toll Free: 877-470-8400
Info@eimcenter.com | www.eimcenter.com

Leonardis Clinic
Abt-Walther-Weg 14-16
83670 Bad Heilbrunn, Germany
Phone: (US contact) 866-631-5444 | Germany: 01149 8046 187 0
Email: info@leonardis-klinik.de | www.leonardisclinic.com

Living Beyond Breast Cancer
Helpline: 888-753-5222 (LBBC)
www.lbbc.org

National Cancer Institute (National Institutes of Health)
NCI Public Inquiries Office
Building 31, Room 10A31
31 Center Drive, MSC 2580
Bethesda, MD 20892-2580 | www.cancer.gov

The National Coalition for Cancer Survivorship
1010 Wayne Avenue, Suite 770
Silver Spring, MD 20910
301-650-9127 | Toll Free: 877-622-7937
info@canceradvocacy.org | www.canceradvocacy.org | www.canscarch.org

Nurses' Health Study
Channing Laboratory
181 Longwood Avenue
Boston, MA 02115
617-525-2279
nhs@channing.harvard.edu | www.nurseshealthstudy.org

The Phyto-Aromatherapy Institute
P.O. Box 3679
South Pasadena, CA 91031
866-44PHYTO (866-447-4986)
mail@phyto-aromatherapy.org | www.phyto-aromatherapy.org

Phyto-Aromatherapy Shoppe & Wellness Center
100 S. Arthur Avenue, Suite 101
Pocatello, ID 83204
Phone: 208-232-5250 | Fax: 208-232-6018

Piny Beverly Hills (wigs and extensions)
8817 West Olympic Blvd., Suite 104
Beverly Hills, CA 90211
Phone: 310-652-6691 | Fax: 310-652-7637
www.pinybeverlyhills.com

Piny Beverly Hills (Sherman Oaks location)
15301 Ventura Blvd., Suite 550, Building B
Sherman Oaks, CA 91403
Phone: 818-784-4247 | Fax: 818-784-4248
www.pinybeverlyhills.com

The Reiki Alliance
204 N. Chestnut Street
Kellogg, ID 83837
208-783-3535
info@reikialliance.com | www.reikialliance.org

Société Française d'Endobiogénie et Médecine (SFEM)
104 Avenue Victor Hugo
75116 Paris, France
sfpa@club-internet.fr

The Susan G. Komen Breast Cancer Foundation
5005 LBJ Freeway, Suite 250
Dallas, TX 75244
972-855-1605 | Helpline: 1-800-I'M AWARE | www.komen.org

Susan Love MD Breast Cancer Research Foundation
P.O. Box 5065
Santa Barbara, CA 93150
805-654-9800 | www.susanlovemdfoundation.org

Time Laboratories
P.O. Box 3243
South Pasadena, CA 91031
Phone: 877-846-3522 | Fax: 888-846-3329
mail@timelabs.com | www.timelabs.com

Suggested Reading

Armstrong, Lance, **"It's Not About The Bike"** A Berkley Book, New York, 2000.

"Breast Cancer, Beyond Convention," Edited by Mary Tagliaferri, M.D., LAc; Isaac Cohen, O.M.D., L.A.c; Debu Tripathy, M.D. Atria Books, New York, London, Toronto, Sydney, Singapore, 2002.

Byrne, Rhonda, **"The Secret."** Atria Books/Beyond Words, November 2006.

Carper, Jean, **"Miracle Cures."** Harper Collins Publishers, New York, 1997.

Cousins, Norman, **"Anatomy of an Illness."** W.W. Norton & Company, Inc., 1979.

Cousins, Norman, **"Head First: The Biology of Hope and the Healing Power of the Human Spirit."** Penguin Books USA, Inc., 1989.

Kraftsow, Gary, **"Yoga For Wellness."** The Penguin Group, New York, 1999.

Lee, John R., M.D., David Zava, Ph.D. and Virginia Hopkins, **"What Your Doctor May Not Tell You About Breast Cancer."** Warner Books, New York, 2002.

Link, John, M.D. **"The Breast Cancer Survival Manual."** Henry Holt and Company, LLC, New York, 1998.

Love, Susan M., M.D. with Karen Lindsey, **"Dr. Susan Love's Breast Book."** Perseus Publishing, Cambridge, MA, 1990.

Plant, Jane A., Ph.D., **"Your Life In Your Hands."** Thomas Dunne Books, New York, 2000, 2001.

Somers, Suzanne, **"The Sexy Years."** Crown Publishing, New York, 2004.

Weiss, Marisa C., M.D. and Ellen Weiss, **"Living Beyond Breast Cancer."** Three Rivers Press, New York, 1997.

Publications in French by Doctors Christian Duraffourd and Jean-Claude Lapraz

"Cahiers de Phytothérapie Clinique" 5 books (Editions Masson 1980–1982) (Clinical Phytotherapy) 4 of them translated in Spanish and Italian.

Summary (7) of the teachings of the year on the first level by the French Society of Phytotherapy and Aromatherapy.

Summary (7) of the congress of Phytotherapy and Aromatherapy.

Publications of the French Society of Phytotherapy and Aromatherapy 1978–2005 (156 leaflets of 70 pages each, for confidential use).

Phytotherapy and Dermatology (Editions Masson 1982 Paris).

Phytotherapy and Aromatherapy: A New Trend in Medicine (1978 Presses de la Renaissance Paris) in collaboration with Dr. Valnet.

Properties and Indications of Small Dosage Oligo-Elements Therapy (Laboratoire des Granions 1988).

Therapeutic Utilization of 84 Medicinal Plants and Essential Oils (Laboratoire Vernin 1989).

Suspensions of Whole Fresh Plants: Clinical Study (Laboratoire Ardeval 1990).

Biological and Clinical Study of Aromatherapy in Relation to 268 Cases of Patients Suffering from Various Infections (Thesis in Medicine by Dr Pierre Lapraz, 1979).

Oncobiology Leaflets (8) Clinique chirurgicale générale et oncologique du Professeur J.Reynier. Hôpital Boucicaut. Paris (1989/1996).

"Medicinal Plants: from Tradition to Science" 97 october (Editor Grancher. Paris)

"Phytotherapy's ABC in Infectious Diseases" (Editor Grancher. 1998 Paris)

"Traité de Phytothérapie Clinique. Endobiogénie et Médecine" (Editions Masson 2002 Paris).

About Doctors Christian Duraffourd and Jean-Claude Lapraz

Doctors Christian Duraffourd and Jean-Claude Lapraz have been active medical practitioners for more than 30 years. They have been involved in the development of clinical phytotherapy (the use of plants or global plant extracts for medicinal purposes) since 1972.

From 1989 to 1996 they served as oncobiologists in the Department of General Surgery and Oncology at Hospital Boucicaut, a leading hospital in Paris, France. They have carried out experimental studies—both in general practice and in a hospital environment—in order to arrive at a rigorous definition of the real therapeutic capabilities of medicinal plants in clinical use.

They have published many books in French, some of which have been translated into Spanish and Italian. They are committed to spreading knowledge about medical phytotherapy within the framework of endobiogénie. The doctors have helped to set up clinical trainings in France, Belgium, Spain, Greece, Italy, Switzerland, Ivory Coast, Tunisia, Mexico, and the United States—all in association with universities or other learned societies in those countries.

They have maintained a close collaboration with official bodies (including the French Ministry of Health and the European Parliament) since 1977, participating in several ministerial commissions. Doctors Duraffourd and Lapraz currently hold numerous offices in professional associations related to phytotherapy.

About the Author

Carol Silverander has had successful careers as an educator, professional photographer, and entrepreneur. She received a degree in Elementary Education from the University of Arizona and a Masters Degree in Photography from Brooks Institute of Photography in Santa Barbara, California.

Carol traveled the world as a photojournalist and documentary photographer, winning many awards. Her work was frequently published and exhibited. She taught photojournalism and social documentary photography at the Univeristy of Arizona in Tucson, and photojournalism at Pima Community College in Tucson.

In 1987 she founded EthnoGraphics, a multicultural greeting card company that went on to acheive national prominence. She sold the company in 2002.

Carol and her husband, Michael, live in Santa Barbara, California and Bend, Oregon with their three dogs: Mattie, Katie and Otis.

Printed in the United States
93659LV00002B/1-16/A